Practice and Principles in Therapeutic Colonoscopy

Dae Kyung Sohn
Editor

Practice and Principles in Therapeutic Colonoscopy

Springer

Editor
Dae Kyung Sohn
National Cancer Center
Goyang-si, Gyeonggi-do
South Korea

ISBN 978-3-662-46551-6 ISBN 978-3-662-46552-3 (eBook)
https://doi.org/10.1007/978-3-662-46552-3

Library of Congress Control Number: 2017954447

Printed on acid-free paper

This Springer imprint is published by Springer Nature
The registered company is Springer-Verlag GmbH Germany
The registered company address is: Heidelberger Platz 3, 14197 Berlin, Germany

Preface

The development of endoscopic technology has increased its therapeutic use over the imaging diagnosis. The common uses of therapeutic colonoscopy are resection of benign and malignant lesions, hemostasis for colorectal bleeding, decompression and recanalization of obstructed bowel, etc. All techniques of therapeutic colonoscopy have been a requirement for an expert endoscopist. This book presents a state-of-the-art knowledge and technique for therapeutic colonoscopy. All technical aspects are covered in detail including indication, instruments, and tips, and the text is complemented by many illustrations. This book will be invaluable in clinical practice for all who are involved or interested in therapeutic colonoscopy.

My deep appreciation goes to professor Jae-Gahb Park and all my colleagues for their unflinching support and encouragement. I'd like to also thank my lovely wife and two children—Jimin and Yuji, who always trust and support me.

Goyang, South Korea — Dae Kyung Sohn
Summer 2017

Contents

Preparation for Therapeutic Colonoscopy

1

Bun Kim

1.1 Introduction

Certain prerequisites should be met before the procedure for a successful and safe therapeutic colonoscopies [1]. First, in terms of patients, sufficient explanation and gaining informed consents in essential. In addition, the patient's concurrent medication and general health condition should be checked. Furthermore, proper sedative and bowel-cleansing agents should be carefully selected for each individual patient (Table 1.1). Second, a colonoscopist should be proficient in therapeutic colonoscopic procedures and well trained assistant including nurses are necessary. Third, the proper systems and instruments including supplies for emergencies should be prepared.

1.2 Patients

1.2.1 Informed Consent for Therapeutic Colonoscopy

Informed consent for therapeutic colonoscopy is obtained in accordance with the informed consent for general colonoscopy. Informed consent is obtained according to hospital or individual center policy.

B. Kim, M.D.
National Cancer Center,
Goyang-si, Gyeonggi-do, South Korea
e-mail: kimbun@ncc.re.kr

Informed consent includes assessment of the competence of the individual to process

Table 1.1 Checklist before therapeutic colonoscopy

Checklist
Current medication
Antiplatelet agent: aspirin, NSAIDs, dipyridamole, thienopyridines (clopidogrel and ticlopidine), GP II/IIIa inhibitors (tirofiban, abciximab, eptifibatide)
Anticoagulant: warfarin, UFH, LMWH
Medication affecting renal function: ACE inhibitor, angiotensin receptor blocker, diuretics, NSAIDs
Patient status
Elderly, childhood, pregnancy, lactation, severe/chronic constipation, diabetes, hypertension, renal dysfunction, congestive heart failure, stroke/dementia, inflammatory bowel disease, lower GI bleeding
Choice of sedative drug
Midazolam, fentanyl, meperidine (pethidine), ketamine, propofol
Diet
Method of diet modulation: clear liquid diet, low residue diet
Duration of diet modulation
Bowel cleansing agent
Choice of bowel cleansing agent: PEG, low volume PEG + ascorbic acid, tablet NaP [32–40], sodium picosulfate + magnesium citrate, additional use of adjunctive agent (magnesium citrate, bisacodyl, etc.)
Intake method of bowel cleansing agent: divided dose regimen, nondivided dose regimen

NSAID nonsteroidal anti-inflammatory drug, *GP* glycoprotein, *UFH* unfractionated heparin, *LMWH* low molecular weight heparin, *ACE* angiotensin converting enzyme, *GI* gastrointestinal, *PEG* polyethylene glycol

D.K. Sohn (ed.), *Practice and Principles in Therapeutic Colonoscopy*,
https://doi.org/10.1007/978-3-662-46552-3_1

Table 1.2 Information to disclose to the average patient

Serious and uncommon risks of colonoscopy, likely to include:
Perforation and bleeding
Could require transfusion or surgery
Serious and uncommon risks associated with colonoscopy and/or the administered anesthesia, which could include:
Cardiac or respiratory complications
Infection (arrhythmia, infarction, aspiration)
Common nonserious risks:
Gas
Bloating
Self-limited discomfort
Intravenous access site complications
Colonoscopy could be an imperfect as a therapeutic procedure:
Possibility of incomplete treatment or recurrence
Possibility of additional surgery or medication for therapy

Table 1.3 Components of the informed consent form

Explanation of the nature and character of the procedure in nontechnical form
Material risks of the procedure
Patient's name
Date and time of consent
Disclaimer of guarantee of success
Identification of the colonoscopist
Consent to allow the physician to modify the procedure for unforeseen circumstances
Acknowledgment of opportunity to ask questions
Consent to disposal of removed tissue
Consent for transmission of results to appropriate parties

information, disclosure of appropriate information necessary to allow an informed decision, and ensuring the plan chosen by the patient is voluntary. The process involves mutual communication and decision-making, not merely the request for a signature on a standardized form that lists complications of a procedure. The four elements of risk that physicians need to consider in providing informed consent are: (1) nature of the risk; (2) magnitude of the risk (seriousness); (3) probability that the risk may occur; (4) imminence of the risk (i.e. post procedure or decades later).

About informed consent for therapeutic colonoscopy, consider information an average patient may want (Table 1.2). Should one mention the possibility of death as a result of the procedure? One study from England reported that a survey of barristers (the English equivalent of plaintiff's attorneys) indicated that serious risks should be mentioned even if as rare as one in a million [2]. Although it is generally legally safer to mention more risks (including very rare risks), there is a potential cost in unnecessarily frightening patients away from beneficial procedures by not adequately conveying the rarity of such an event.

In process of consent, the colonoscopist must ensure that the patient is competent to understand the information disclosed. Note that the medical literature contains information indicating that ordinarily competent older patients may be temporarily unable to adequately comprehend information when hospitalized with a serious illness. Having a family member present may be useful to ensure adequate consent or at least reduce the likelihood of successful consent challenge later. Informational materials may be given to the patient to facilitate understanding of the procedure. Appropriate institutional forms should be signed and witnessed, and a statement written or dictated as part of the colonoscopy note indicating that informed consent has been obtained. It is best if the witness to consent is a family member or friend, since this implies that the witness believes the patient capable of consent, and is also there to help in the process. If a member of staff witnesses the consent, it is best if this is not the person obtaining the consent or helping perform the procedure. If an issue comes to trial and those in the procedure room are named as defendants, their testimony witnessing the adequacy of consent may appear biased.

The standard core elements of informed consent (Table 1.3) include the nature and character of the procedure (preferably in nontechnical terms), the material risks of the procedure, the likely benefits, and the potential alternatives (including no treatment). Most consent forms will also include the patient's name, date and time of consent, disclaimer of guarantee of success, identification of staff who will perform the

Table 1.4 Exceptions to informed consent

Emergencies
Implied consent
Patient waives right to informed consent
Therapeutic privilege
Legal mandates

procedure, consent to allow the physician to modify the procedure for unforeseen circumstances, an acknowledgment that the patient has been given the opportunity to ask questions which have been answered, consent to disposal of removed organs, and, with new privacy concerns and regulations, consent for transmission of the results to appropriate parties.

In colonoscopies, the exceptions to informed consents could be applied with caution (Table 1.4). In an emergency situation, a health-care provider may treat the patient without obtaining consent; consent is presumed, or "implied" in legal parlance. The definition of emergency may vary in different jurisdictions, but the principles of imminent harm by failure of prompt treatment can be applied. This issue is less likely to arise with colonoscopy. Further, attempting even a limited consent with a conscious patient is worthwhile if it will not unduly delay emergency treatment.

Patients are able to waive their right to informed consent. However, they must know they have the right to information necessary to make an informed decision. Thus when a colonoscopy patient says "You're the doctor, you decide what is best," the careful doctor may accept that responsibility but will first inform the patient of the right to information and decision-making.

Therapeutic privilege allows physicians to withhold information they generally must disclose, based upon the physician's perception that disclosure will be harmful to the patient. However, this is a disfavored exception; there is concern that it may be used as an excuse for not informing patients. Unless there is clear and convincing evidence of psychologic fragility, it would be best to ignore this exception.

The ethical and legal requirement to obtain informed consent prior to performing colonoscopy derives from the concept of personal (patient) autonomy. The competent patient, after receiving appropriate disclosure of the material risks of the procedure, understanding those risks, the benefits, and the alternative approaches, makes a voluntary and uncoerced informed decision to proceed. This is a basic ethical obligation in the practice of medicine. It should be a communication tool that cements the provider–patient relationship. It functions as a risk-management tool, transferring known standard procedural risks to the patient who has understood and accepted the premise that even competently performed colonoscopy has risks. The procedural elements involved in obtaining consent include a discussion of material risks, acknowledge of who gives and obtains consent, the scope of consent, exceptions to consent, witnessing and documentation of consent, and the use of educational materials and consent forms.

Consent is a mutual process, which occurs after appropriate disclosure, with time for answering questions, in an uncoerced process. In open-access colonoscopy, the patient has not met the colonoscopist prior to the decision to proceed with colonoscopy, prior to having undergone preparation for the procedure, or in some cases prior to arriving in the procedure room with an intravenous line in place.

1.2.2 Modulation of Medication

As the elderly population grows, more patients receiving medications such as aspirin, anticoagulants, and nonsteroidal anti-inflammatory drugs (NSAIDs), are being referred to endoscopists for therapeutic colonoscopy. For patient's convenience, polypectomy is often performed as soon as a polyp is detected to avoid another bowel preparation. Therefore, if the patient's concurrent medication increases the risk of bleeding after polypectomy, this should be considered before the colonoscopy. The patients in whom discontinuation of the antithrombotic agent poses only a low risk may stop their medication during the periendoscopic period [3–5]. However, a careful evaluation is needed in cases when discontinuation of the antithrombotic agent is associated with a high risk of adverse effects [3–5]. A previous study showed that the use of aspirin or clopidogrel alone was not related to higher rates of post-polypectomy bleeding [6].

The management of the medications needs to be considered during the periendoscopic period in patients receiving anticoagulant agents such as warfarin, unfractionated heparin (UFH), and low molecular weight heparin (LMWH), and anti-platelet agents such as aspirin, NSAIDs, dipyridamole, thienopyridines (clopidogrel and ticlopidine), and glycoprotein II/IIIa (GP II/IIIa) inhibitors (tirofiban, abciximab, and eptifibatide) [3–5]. The management is based on the assessment of the procedure-related bleeding risk and potential thromboembolic risks related to the discontinuation of the medication [3–5].

Aspirin and/or NSAIDs are recommended to be continued during all endoscopic procedures, and clinicians may discontinue aspirin and/or NSAIDs for 5–7 days before the high-risk procedures such as polypectomy and endoscopic submucosal dissection [3–5]. In patients with a vascular stent or acute coronary syndrome, clopidogrel or ticlopidine may be withheld for 7–10 days before the endoscopy, provided that a minimum recommended period after the corresponding treatment has passed, and aspirin could be continued [3–5]. If clopidogrel or ticlopidine is used for other indications, these medications could be continued for low-risk procedures such as diagnostic colonoscopy including biopsy. However, they need to be discontinued for 7–10 days before high-risk procedures. Anticoagulant (warfarin) discontinuation is recommended in patients with a low risk of thromboembolic events [3–5] (Table 1.5).

Continuation of anticoagulation by switching to LM-WH or UFH is recommended in the periendoscopic period in patients with higher risks of thromboembolic complications [3–5] (Table 1.5). In patients with a high risk of thromboembolic events, UFH or LMWH needs to be restarted as soon as possible, and warfarin can be restarted on the day of the procedure without a significant danger of bleeding [3–5]. In patients with a low risk of thromboembolic events, warfarin may be restarted on the evening after the endoscopy without a high risk of postprocedural bleeding [5].

Table 1.5 Conditions for the risk of thromboembolic events

High-risk condition	Atrial fibrillation associated valvular heart disease, prosthetic valve, active congestive heart failure, left ventricular ejection fraction <35%, history of a thromboembolic event, hypertension, diabetes mellitus or age > 75 years
	Mechanical valve in the mitral position
	Mechanical valve in any position and previous thromboembolic event
	Recently (<1 year) placed coronary stent Acute coronary syndrome
	Nonstented percutaneous coronary intervention after myocardial infarction
Low-risk condition	Uncomplicated or paroxysmal nonvalvular atrial fibrillation
	Bioprosthetic valve
	Mechanical valve in the aortic position
	Deep vein thrombosis

In patients with acute GI bleeding receiving an anticoagulant or antiplatelet agent, this medication is recommended to be withheld until hemostasis is achieved [5].

1.2.3 Endoscopic Sedation

The purposes of procedure-related sedation include safe and effective management of pain and anxiety in addition to acquirement of a proper degree of memory loss and decreased awareness. Currently, there is no standard regimen regarding sedation in GI endoscopy [7]. The choice of sedation may differ depending on the endoscopist's preferences and the type of planned procedure. In special conditions such as obesity, pregnancy, advanced age, and chronic lung, liver or renal disease, special considerations and precautions are required regarding the dose adjustment and choice of sedative drugs [7, 8].

Midazolam is considered the benzodiazepine of choice as it provides a shorter duration of action with a better pharmacokinetic profile than diazepam [7, 8]. Pethidine and fentanyl are the most popular [7, 8]. Reversal drugs for endoscopic sedative drugs consist of flumazenil and naloxone [8] Flumazenil, a benzodiazepine antagonist, reverses the respiratory and sedative effects of benzodiazepine [8]. Naloxone, a pure mu-opioid antagonist, reverses both the respiratory and analgesic effects of opioids [7, 8].

Unsedated endoscopic procedures are recommended for elderly patients or patients with the risk of cardiopulmonary dysfunction.

The use of propofol for sedation during diagnostic and therapeutic procedures is increasing as it enhances the quality of upper GI endoscopy by increasing the patient's acceptance of the procedure and the diagnostic accuracy [9]. In addition, it has satisfactory sedative, hypnotic, antiemetic, and amnesic properties, as well as a rapid onset of action and a short recovery profile [7, 8]. Its use is preferred in patients with advanced liver disease because of its short biologic half-life resulting in a low risk of hepatic encephalopathy [8]. With regard to side effects, propofol may induce cardiopulmonary events. It can cause a dose-dependent decrease in cardiac contractility leading to a decrease in cardiac output, systemic vascular resistance, and arterial pressure [7, 8]. In addition, it may be associated with serious adverse events such as respiratory depression, airway obstruction, and death [7, 8]. Unfortunately, there is no pharmacological antagonist for this compound [7, 8]. In a prolonged and potentially uncomfortable endoscopic procedure, intravenous midazolam along with propofol for sedation has been reported to be more effective than intravenous midazolam alone, without differences in the safety [10].

Meperidine (category B) followed by small doses of midazolam (category D) as needed is recommended for moderate sedation in endoscopic procedures during pregnancy [11]. Breastfeeding may be continued after fentanyl (category C) or propofol (category B) administration in lactating patients after sufficient recovery from general anesthesia. Infants should not be breastfed for at least 4 h after midazolam is administered to the mother [11].

Patient's age, inpatient status, higher American Society of Anesthesia grade (Table 1.6), routine use of oxygen, and trainee participation were associated with a higher incidence of unplanned cardiopulmonary events during GI endoscopy under conscious sedation [12].

Table 1.6 Definition of ASA status

Class 1	Patient has no organic, physiological, biochemical, or psychiatric disturbance. The pathological process for which the operation is to be performed is localized and does not entail systemic disturbance
Class 2	Mild to moderate systemic disturbance caused either by the condition to be treated surgically or by other pathophysiological processes
Class 3	Severe, systemic disturbance or disease from whatever cause, even though it may not be possible to define the degree of disability with finality
Class 4	Severe systemic disorders that are already life threatening, not always correctable by operation
Class 5	The moribund patient who has little chance of survival but is submitted to operation in desperation

1.2.4 Diet

Although dietary modifications alone are not sufficient for preparation for colonoscopy, they have proven to be effective when conducted together with mechanical cleansing [13]. For dietary regimens, clear liquids and low-residue diets are recommended for 1–4 days before colonoscopy [13, 14]. Patients are allowed to have water, clear soup, clear fruit juice without pulp, coffee or tea without milk, and sport drinks on the clear liquid diet [14]. In addition, patients may have white rice, white rice cakes, refined noodles or pasta, vegetable juices, grapes without skin and seeds, peaches without skins and seeds, watermelon without seeds, well-cooked potatoes without skin, tender meat, fish, chicken, and eggs on the low-residue diet [14]. Patients are forbidden to have high-fiber foods such as brown rice, whole grains, raw and dried fruits, seeds, nuts, and multigrain bread [14]. Prolonged dietary restrictions may also be an important factor for better colon preparation, but they could lead to lower compliance [13]. Nevertheless, prolonged fiber restriction with liquid diet needs to be suggested in cases of severe constipation [15]. Furthermore, a study suggested that the fiber-free diet is more effective than the clear liquid diet if it is combined with the use of polyethylene glycol (PEG) electrolyte solution on the day before colonoscopy [16].

1.2.5 Bowel Preparation

The ideal preparation for colonoscopy needs to satisfy the requirement of emptying the colon of all solid or liquid materials in a rapid fashion with no gross or histological changes in the colonic mucosa. Additionally, shifts in fluids or electrolytes, patient discomfort, and cost should be kept to the minimum [17].

PEG-electrolyte lavage solution is the most frequently prescribed bowel-cleansing agent. As it is a nonabsorbable solution, it passes through the bowel without net absorption or secretion, and significant fluid or electrolyte shifts do not occur [13]. Therefore, PEG is considered safer than stimulant laxative/sodium phosphate (NaP) in patients with fluid or electrolyte imbalance [13]. It is preferred in patients with renal insufficiency, congestive heart failure, or liver failure [13] The drawbacks of this agent are that it should be diluted in a large volume of water (up to 4 L) to reach the desired cathartic effect and it's unpalatable taste despite flavoring, which leads to poor compliance [13]. Sulfate-free PEG (SF-PEG) was developed to improve the taste and smell of the PEG solution by decreasing the potassium concentration, increasing the chloride concentration, and eliminating sodium sulfate [13]. SF-PEG is considered to be comparable to PEG in safety, effectiveness, and tolerance, but it still requires consumption of 4 L of the diluted agent [13]. Aqueous NaP is no longer prescribed, as it may cause significant fluid and electrolyte shifts resulting in renal failure; however, NaP tablets are still available. Adjunctive agents are used to enhance the cleansing efficacy of bowel preparation conducted by the main purgative regimens such as PEG, as well as to reduce the volume of fluid that needs to be taken to achieve a cathartic effect [18]. Ascorbic acid, which is not completely absorbed and remains in the colonic lumen, exerts an osmotic effect and is used with a smaller quantity of PEG [19, 20]. Low-volume PEG solutions with ascorbic acid have been reported to be comparable to high-volume PEG solutions in efficacy and tolerability by the patients [19, 20]. Magnesium salts that show a synergic effect through their osmogenic properties are often used with picosulfate, a prodrug that is metabolized to a peristalsis-enhancing stimulant within the bowel lumen [21]. The regimen with sodium picosulfate and magnesium citrate is gradually accepted as a major bowel-cleansing regimen based on its efficacy and safety profiles [22]. Other adjuncts such as bisacodyl, senna, and metoclopramide have been reported to have the advantage of reducing the volume of the solution required for bowel cleansing; however, their exact efficacies and safety profiles remain to be established [13, 18, 23].

A meta-analysis found that a divided-dose PEG solution regimen (initial 2–3 L is given the night prior to the colonoscopy and the remaining 1–2 L on the morning of the procedure) improves the quality of bowel preparation, increases patient compliance, and reduces the incidence of nausea that leads patients to discontinue bowel preparation when compared with full-dose PEG [13, 24].

The quality of bowel preparation may be influenced by the interval between the end of the preparation procedure and the start of colonoscopy [25]. It is suggested that colonoscopy needs to be performed within 7 h from the start of PEG intake and 4 h from the end of PEG intake to improve the quality of bowel preparation [25]. If colonoscopy is scheduled in the afternoon, bowel preparation may be carried out on the same day, resulting in better feasibility, safety, and effectiveness, as well as fewer adverse events, and leading to patients' preference [25, 26].

Elderly patients tend to show higher rates of inadequate colon cleansing for colonoscopy [27]. A dietary restriction is helpful, with clear liquids and low-residue diets for 1–4 days prior to the colonoscopy [15]. Moreover, cleansing by PEG consumption <5 h prior to colonoscopy is efficient [15].

In patients with severe constipation, a longer period of staying on a liquid diet, application of

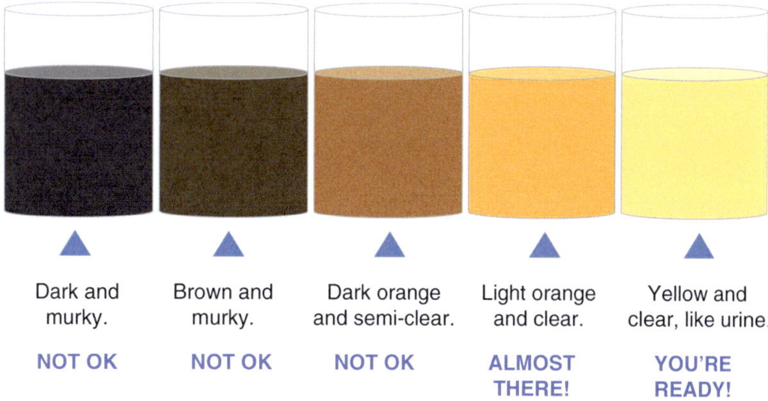

Fig. 1.1 Sample page from booklet addressing importance of bowel preparation quality: Provides instructions for how to interpret stool effluent to help ensure high-quality preparation [33]

alternating bowel-cleansing agents, use of an adjunctive laxative, and use of a double dose of the PEG solution are recommended for successful bowel preparation, as they have increased colon transit time and may be resistant to laxatives [15].

Patients with stroke may have difficulties swallowing, and patients with dementia may have difficulties taking large amounts of fluid [15]. The bowel preparation solution may be administered directly into the stomach or duodenum through an esophagogastroduodenoscope using a water irrigation pump or nasogastric tube [13, 15, 28].

In patients with lower GI bleeding, adequate bowel preparation may be beneficial for the identification of the bleeding source [15]. If the amount of bleeding is suspected to be small, bowel preparation using PEG solution may be helpful. However, enema is preferred if the bleeding source is presumed to be within the rectal area, or the amount of bleeding is suspected to be severe [15, 29].

Appropriate bowel preparation is closely related to the compliance of the patient to the preparation instructions. Therefore, patients' understanding of colonoscopy and bowel preparation may influence the outcome of the procedure. One study suggested that non-compliance with bowel preparation instructions and lower education level were independent risk factors for poor bowel preparation [30]. Education of patients is considered a very important factor to ensure compliance before colonoscopy, and many studies have suggested diverse education programs that have resulted in apparent increases in patient compliance [31–35]. Nurse-delivered education with brochures, an educational pamphlet, a novel patient educational booklet, and cartoon visual aids were suggested to be effective in increasing the quality of bowel preparation [31–34] (Fig. 1.1).

1.3 Endoscopist

1.3.1 Qualified in Therapeutic Colonoscopy

Therapeutic colonoscopy is a complex endoscopic procedure that involves therapeutic maneuvers such as polypectomy. Colonoscopy has significant potential not only to benefit patients but also to cause adverse outcomes due to incomplete or failed therapies, and complications.

Traditionally, the assessment of competence has relied on tallying total numbers of procedures performed or subjective evaluation by a proctor. The use of threshold procedure numbers at which competence may be globally assessed provides only a rough guide for evaluation of competence.

Suggested objective performance criteria for the evaluation of technical skills in gastrointestinal endoscopy are listed in Table 1.7 [36]. It has been proposed that expert endoscopists should be

Table 1.7 Suggested objective performance criteria for the evaluation of technical skills in gastrointestinal endoscopy as proposed by the American Society for Gastrointestinal Endoscopy [36]

Procedure	Performance criteria
Colonoscopy	Intubation of splenic flexure
	Intubation of cecum
	Intubation of terminal ileum (desirable skill)
Polypectomy	Successful performance
All procedures	Accurate recognition of normal and abnormal findings
	Development of appropriate endoscopic/medical treatment in response to endoscopic findings

Table 1.8 Recommendations of the American Society for Gastrointestinal Endoscopy for minimum number of procedures before competency can be assessed [37]

Standard procedure	Number of cases required
Total colonoscopy	100
Snare polypectomy	20[a]
Flexible sigmoidoscopy	25

[a]Included in total number

expected to perform at a technical success level of 95–100% [36]. The available data support as reasonable the standard of 80–90% technical success before trainees are deemed competent in a specific skill.

Recommendations of various organizations on minimum numbers of procedures required to achieve competence Medical societies have issued position papers regarding how much training is required to achieve competence in colonoscopy.

Official recommendations of organizations have included those of the American Society for Gastrointestinal Endoscopy (ASGE), which recommends a minimum of 100 colonoscopies to achieve competence [37] (Table 1.8); the British Society of Gastroenterology, which recommends 100 colonoscopies; the Conjoint Committee for Recognition of Training in Gastrointestinal Endoscopy of Australia, which recommends 100 colonoscopies; and the European Diploma of Gastroenterology, which suggests 100 colonoscopies. In contrast to gastroenterology-oriented societies, other specialties have often suggested that much lower numbers would be adequate; for example, the Society of American Gastrointestinal Endoscopic Surgery (SAGES) has recommended 25 procedures. Recently, at the urging of the ASGE, SAGES has agreed to eliminate suggested numbers of procedures (personal communication from ASGE). The American Academy of Family Practice has endorsed "short courses" during which trainees perform an average of less than ten supervised procedures [38].

It is clear that performance of a minimum number of procedures, although a prerequisite for acquiring skill, does not guarantee competence. Because subjective assessment of competence by a proctor is often inaccurate, objective assessment of performance at endoscopy is necessary to assess accurately the competence of an individual. Such objective performance data are useful not only in training but also for credentialing, obtaining hospital privileges, and perhaps even allowing patients and healthcare providers to choose their physicians.

1.4 System and Instruments

1.4.1 Training Colonoscopy Assistant

A trained gastrointestinal assistant is a necessary and important part of the endoscopy team. During the procedure, the assistant works closely with the endoscopist, often preparing the necessary equipment in advance of the physician's request, and anticipates the next set of actions. However, the intraprocedure part of the assistant's task is only one part of the overall responsibility. Other duties of the gastrointestinal assistant include: preparation of the room, ordering supplies, speaking with the patient and allaying apprehensions, cleaning and maintaining the equipment, coordinating outgoing specimens and incoming reports with the pathology laboratory, keeping track of narcotics and their proper requisition.

Because of the complex nature of the therapeutic colonoscopy and the multiple elements that must be learned, proficiency of the assistant and efficiency of the endoscopy unit mandates that proper training is required in order to be a gastrointestinal assistant.

The role and responsibility of the assistant during colonoscopy varies according to level of licensure. The nurse and associate must function within these prescribed guidelines and hospital or facility policy.

When a patient is scheduled for the procedure, instructions for colon preparation are supplied. The patient's medical history is important in the decision of which method is used for cleansing the colon. It is at this time that the teaching process is begun. Brochures are often helpful for this initial contact, as it gives the patient a statement to take home and read in a less stressful surrounding [39].

After arrival at the endoscopy center for the procedure, the patient is escorted and instructed to change into a procedure gown. It is critical to obtain a basic medical history, including allergies, current medications, and a record of past surgical procedures.

Physical limitations and psychological issues should be included and addressed. Of special note are any medical conditions that put the patient at increased risk of developing a complication related to sedation. These include severe cardiac, pulmonary, renal or central nervous system disorders, and obesity, sleep apnea, pregnancy, and drug or alcohol abuse. The medication list should include all drugs that the patient is taking on a routine or PRN basis. This includes prescription drugs, over-the-counter medications, vitamins, and herbs. The endoscopist should be notified if the patient is taking medications that affect coagulation including warfarin, aspirin, nonsteroidal antiinflammatory drugs, and ginko. The assistant should be aware of possible adverse medication interaction with agents used for sedation, analgesia. Examples include benzodiazepines, opioids, psychoactive drugs, and monoamine oxidase inhibitors. Meperidine should not be given to a patient who has taken a monoamine oxidase inhibitor within 2–3 weeks as coma, severe hypertension, hypotension, respiratory depression, convulsions, malignant hyperpyrexia, and death may occur. There can also be a potentiating effect with the administration of any narcotic agent.

The effectiveness of the colon preparation should be established during the interview. The nurse should ask the patient what preparation he/she took and for a description of the last results. If there is a questionable or poor result, the endoscopist should be notified for a decision to perform the procedure, give an enema, or reschedule after re-prepping the patient.

1.4.2 Setting Up the Room

The equipment should be turned on and all operating systems initiated. Water bottles should be sterilized or high-level disinfected daily. If high-level disinfectant is used, a thorough rinse with sterile water should be performed to remove chemical residue. Water bottles should then be filled with sterile water to the level indicated, and the top secured and positioned according to manufacturer's instructions.

The assistant should check the procedure room for the availability of supplies (medication, accessories, biopsy forceps, specimen containers, etc.) and test all equipment for functionality. Accessories for colonoscopy are used for snare polypectomy, tissue sampling, endoscopic mucosal resection, object retrieval, size measurement, marking, image enhancement, hemostasis, ablation, and stenting. In addition, technologic advances in the design of the clipping, looping and banding devices have made their use in the colon relatively user-friendly and they should be part of the available accessories in all endoscopy units undertaking colonoscopy. Their application is mainly in the prevention and treatment of complications such as postpolypectomy hemorrhage. Appropriate use allows safer and more effective colonoscopic therapy. The colonoscope should be tested to assure that air and water channels are working. Lubricant should be ready for the endoscopist to use for rectal examination and lubrication of the instrument prior to insertion.

1.4.3 Monitoring and Sedation

There is a critical nature to the assignment of monitoring the patient who is receiving sedation and analgesia. For very ill patients and/or the complex procedures, a second nurse or associate is required to assist the physician while a registered nurse concentrates on monitoring the patient [40].

Basic life support is a standard requirement for all healthcare workers. In some centers, advanced cardiac life support is required for licensed personnel. Emergency equipment should be available and staff should be familiar with this equipment and its location. Several sizes of oral airways, and mask and bag equipment for respiratory support should be readily available.

There should be immediate access to an emergency cart with a defibrillator, emergency drugs, and intubation equipment. For a colonoscopy, most patients receive medication for sedation and analgesia. Because of this, additional training regarding the role of staff during administration of these medications may be required. Critical are the knowledge of correct doses, possible cumulative effects, interactions with other medications, and the role of monitoring the patient for respiratory depression. Staff should also be familiar with pharmacologic antagonists for opioids and benzodiazepines. The patient is escorted to the procedure room by the assistant and baseline vital signs are obtained.

The patient's vital signs will be monitored during the procedure. This monitoring should include blood pressure, pulse, and pulse oximetry, the patient's level of pain and response to the procedure. Ventilatory function should be observed visually throughout the procedure.

This information should be recorded in the patient's record. Automatic monitoring devices may enhance the ability to accurately assess the patient, but are no substitute for the watchful, educated assessment by a registered nurse [41, 42].

Depending on center policy, ongoing interval blood pressure measurement, and continuous heart rate and pulse oximetry readings are measured. Recommendations from the American Society of Anesthesiologists (ASA) include that the type and amount of medication administered, length of the procedure, and the general condition of the patient should be the factors to determine frequency of measurement. At a minimum, these measurements should be obtained and recorded prior to the start of the procedure, after administration of sedative/analgesic agents, completion of the procedure, during initial recovery, and at the time of discharge. Regular readings and recording of vital signs should be incorporated into the policy of the endoscopy unit, such as: obtain blood pressure, pulse, and pulse oximetry readings before the procedure, every 5 min during the procedure, and in the immediate recovery phase. Cardiac monitoring is done if the patient has a history of cardiac disease. When the patient is transferred to the recovery area, blood pressure, pulse, and pulse oximetry should be measured on arrival and at specified intervals, such as every 15 min, for a minimum of 30 min, until discharge. Excessive sedation may result in cardiac or respiratory depression. These symptoms must be rapidly recognized, reported to the endoscopist, and treated to avoid the risk of hypoxic brain damage, cardiac arrest, or death. The person assigned to monitor the patient should be situated facing the patient and only assist with minor interruptible tasks. A second assistant should be present for sick patients and complicated procedures [40].

If hypoxemia occurs during sedation, supplemental oxygen is to be administered immediately. The use of capnography via a nasal cannula with a CO_2 sensor in addition to pulse oximetry to monitor for hypoxia appears to be superior to close observation of the patient during the procedure [43, 44].

Despite an excellent overall safety record, cardiopulmonary complications, likely due to sedative and analgesic medications are believed to account for 50–60% of procedure-related morbidity and mortality, respectively [45].

1.4.4 The Assistant During the Procedure

Staff should be in personal protective equipment before the procedure is started. The patient is assisted to the left lateral position with knees bent

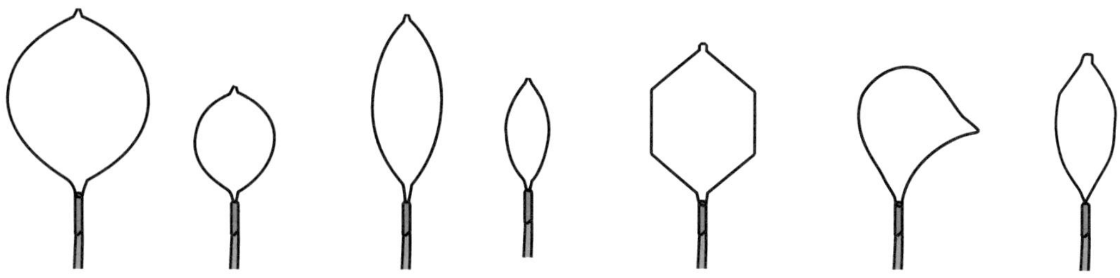

Fig. 1.2 Polypectomy snares. Snares differ in loop diameter, shape, and filament diameter. After it is embedded in the mucosa, the pointed tip can act as a fulcrum (Practical Colonoscopy Jerome D. Waye et al. Wiley Blackwell)

for the start of the procedure. Many endoscopists find that there are benefits to repositioning the patient during the procedure.

The patient may be asked to turn to supine, right lateral, and occasionally to a prone position. Although it is difficult to have an oversedated, ill, or elderly patient change position, most patients can change position with minimal assistance and verbal cues. The assistant must be aware of multiple safety issues when repositioning the patient. The patient's position in relation to the edge of the cart or table must be carefully observed. To prevent injury to the patient or damage to equipment, attachments such as monitoring wires, grounding pads, and oxygen tubing should be checked after any position change is made.

An adequate number of specimen containers and labels with appropriate patient information should be available before the start of the colonoscopy. The assistant must be observant during the procedure so that the.

Both the patient and equipment can be prepared as the procedure progresses. When a polyp requiring electrocautery is encountered, the grounding pad can be applied to the patient and an appropriate snare chosen (Fig. 1.2).

Biopsy forceps or other equipment can also be readied when need is anticipated.

Operation of a snare: Since there are a number of sizes and shapes of snares available, the choice is made by the endoscopist according to the size and location of the polyp in the colon. The assistant usually opens and closes the snare as requested. Snare cutting is dependent upon a combination of mechanical forces of the wire closing against the plastic sheath and the use of high-frequency current, which is produced by an electrocautery machine. The sheath may compress during snare closure so that the tip of the snare, which withdrew into the sheath when tested outside the patient, cannot be fully withdrawn once around a polyp because the sheath has shortened with compression. This may preclude complete resection and cause an impacted snare. To avoid this problem, verify that the tip of the wire snare retracts at least 15 mm into the sheath prior to polypectomy.

The assistant should be familiar with each electrosurgical unit being used in the endoscopy center. In some cases, current output may vary according to unit or manufacturer. Instructions and use of settings specific to the units available in the department should be readily available for training and reference purposes.

If an electrical grounding pad is used, the usual placement is on the upper thigh or lower trunk, whichever is the largest tissue mass. To ensure complete contact with the patient's skin, the chosen area should be dry and as free from hair as possible. If a polyp is to be removed, a specimen trap should be placed between the scope and the suction tubing to retrieve any tissue suctioned through the scope (Fig. 1.3). The active cord is connected between the snare and the electrosurgical unit and the dial is set as appropriate per manufacturer's directions, unit policy, and by the endoscopist's preference. Electrical currents that have a pure cutting effect are usually not employed for colonoscopic polypectomy.

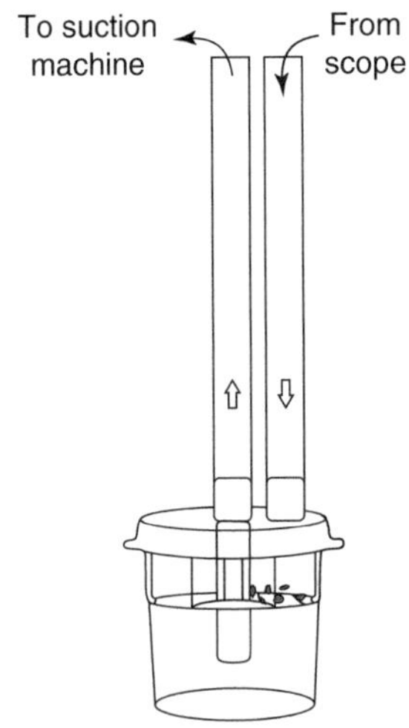

Fig. 1.3 Polyp retrieval trap. A compartmented trap permits capture of polyp from different areas of the colon. Even samples taken by biopsy forceps will be caught within the small grid that collects polyps

Electro-coagulation current alone may be used or a blend of cut and coagulation may be applied. The activation pedal for the unit is placed in position for ready access to the endoscopist.

During polypectomy, the endoscopist will position the sheath and give the order to open the snare. The assistant will extend the loop and the endoscopist will position the loop around the polyp. The assistant should be sure that the electrocautery unit is turned on before use and ensure that the active cord is securely connected. Upon the direction to close the snare, it is important for the assistant to close the snare slowly while maintaining continuous communication with the endoscopist. While visualizing the polyp and feeling for resistance, the assistant will close the loop on the snare slowly until tension is felt and the loop can be seen to be in the proper position. When ready for electrocautery, the endoscopist will depress the foot pedal and give the direction to close.

If saline injection is used to lift the polyp tissue from the mucosal wall, an injection needle and normal saline for should be available. One or two 10 cc syringes should be prepared depending on the size and number of polyps. The normal saline should be drawn up and, depending on the endoscopist's preference, a drop or two of methylene blue can also be drawn up in the syringe. The advantage of using the methylene blue is that the blush of the tissue as well as the translucent color can identify the margins of the polyp. Whenever methylene blue is used during a procedure, the patient must be advised that their urine may turn green and there may be a color change in their stool as the medication is excreted. Advising them of the possible color change before discharge will prevent a panicked phone call regarding the strange color of their urine.

The severed polyp may be retrieved in several ways. If a biopsy forceps or hot biopsy forceps are used, the tissue is removed with the forceps. Small polyps can be readily retrieved by suction into a small capture bottle (trap) attached to the main suction plug of the instrument. For larger polyps removed with a snare, suction can be used to secure it to the end of the scope. The polyp can be resnared to carry it out of the colon, or an entrapment or retrieval device such as a basket or tripod grasper can be used. For multiple polyps, each polyp specimen should be placed in an individual container with the site clearly identified in addition to the patient information. The ability to keep all specimens in their proper order (size, location, method of removal) is aided by keeping a written log of each event as it occurs.

Colorectal bleeding: When a bleeding site is encountered, several items of equipment must be available for immediate use. Review of skills on a regular basis is essential, especially with devices that are used on an irregular basis. Devices or instruments available include injection needles, bipolar probes, detachable snares, clip devices, argon ionized coagulator, laser and heater probes. As technology changes and advances, other instruments may be available in the future.

Epinephrine 1:10,000 is often the hemostatic agent of choice. Most sites are injected with 1–2 mL as instructed by the endoscopist.

A detachable snare may be used in the event that the area bleeding is clearly identified, such as a polyp stalk following transection. The snare is tightened on the bleeding area and when secure it is detached from the device and left in place. After healing occurs, the snare sloughs off and is passed with the patient's stool.

There are several options available when using a bipolar probe. There are 7Fr and 10Fr sizes available with or without a needle for injection. Having the needle built in is helpful when that need is anticipated, but can be more difficult to deploy than a standard injection needle.

It is ideal to have an additional staff member available during and after these complex procedures to assist with equipment and disinfecting the procedure area following the procedure. This enables close monitoring of the patient and the effectiveness of interventions, as well as efficient room turnover between procedures.

1.4.5 Protective Gear for Therapeutic Colonoscopy

Blood is not the only source of exposure to potentially infectious materials. Other potentially infectious materials include, but are not limited to, human body fluids such as saliva, peritoneal fluid, stool, and unfixed human tissue [46].

It is possible for almost every employee of an endoscopy center to have occupational exposure to blood or other potentially infectious material. All nurses and associates are regularly exposed to these materials and even ward clerks or secretaries may be exposed on occasion when they handle specimens.

Protective gear should be universally used to provide a physical barrier for staff during interactions with patients when there is a potential for exposure to infectious and toxic substances. Because the same measures are used in every case, body substance precautions protect the healthcare worker from unrecognized or asymptomatic cases of infectious diseases as well as recognized or symptomatic cases.

Protective gear should include a gown, eye protection, a face mask or shield if splash is anticipated, and gloves for every event which presents the possibility of exposure. Radiation and laser protection should be provided if these therapeutic measures are needed.

Semipermeable gowns can be used if excessive splash is not anticipated. Non-permeable gowns in either plastic or treated fabric are available to protect staff members from any type of splash.

Eye protection, either safety goggles/glasses, or face shields should provide adequate protection without restricting movement or vision. The equipment should be provided by the employer and should be durable, easy to clean and disinfect. Staff members should keep safety equipment clean and in good repair.

Gloves should meet the need of the staff member and the patient. Any sensitivity to latex should be noted and taken seriously as anaphylaxis can occur and is a lifethreatening event. Gloves should be removed immediately following the procedure or in the event there is a possibility of a break in the surface integrity. Hands should be washed immediately after gloves or personal protective equipment are removed. In accordance with sound occupational health principles, employee training should occur prior to the time that the employee is placed in a situation where exposure could occur. Training must be provided at the time of the initial assignment or job change that causes exposure and must be repeated annually [46].

References

1. Rex DK, Bond JH, Winawer S, Levin TR, Burt RW, Johnson DA, et al. Quality in the technical performance of colonoscopy and the continuous quality improvement process for colonoscopy: recommendations of the U.S. Multi-Society Task Force on Colorectal Cancer. Am J Gastroenterol. 2002;97(6):1296–308.
2. Ward B, Shah S, Kirwan P, Mayberry JF. Issues of consent in colonoscopy: if a patient says 'stop' should we continue? J R Soc Med. 1999;92(3):132–3.
3. Veitch AM, Baglin TP, Gershlick AH, Harnden SM, Tighe R, Cairns S, et al. Guidelines for the management of anticoagulant and antiplatelet therapy in patients undergoing endoscopic procedures. Gut. 2008;57(9):1322–9.
4. Boustiere C, Veitch A, Vanbiervliet G, Bulois P, Deprez P, Laquiere A, et al. Endoscopy and antiplatelet agents. European Society of Gastrointestinal Endoscopy (ESGE) guideline. Endoscopy. 2011;43(5):445–61.
5. ASGE Standards of Practice Committee, Anderson MA, Ben-Menachem T, Gan SI, Appalaneni V, Banerjee S, et al. Management of antithrombotic agents for endoscopic procedures. Gastrointest Endosc. 2009;70(6):1060–70.

6. Singh M, Mehta N, Murthy UK, Kaul V, Arif A, Newman N. Postpolypectomy bleeding in patients undergoing colonoscopy on uninterrupted clopidogrel therapy. Gastrointest Endosc. 2010;71(6):998–1005.
7. Triantafillidis JK, Merikas E, Nikolakis D, Papalois AE. Sedation in gastrointestinal endoscopy: current issues. World J Gastroenterol. 2013;19(4):463–81.
8. Amornyotin S. Sedation and monitoring for gastrointestinal endoscopy. World J Gastrointest Endosc. 2013;5(2):47–55.
9. Meining A, Semmler V, Kassem AM, Sander R, Frankenberger U, Burzin M, et al. The effect of sedation on the quality of upper gastrointestinal endoscopy: an investigator-blinded, randomized study comparing propofol with midazolam. Endoscopy. 2007;39(4):345–9.
10. Kim YS, Kim MH, Jeong SU, Lee BU, Lee SS, Park DH, et al. Comparison between midazolam used alone and in combination with propofol for sedation during endoscopic retrograde cholangiopancreatography. Clin Endosc. 2014;47(1):94–100.
11. ASGE Standard of Practice Committee, Shergill AK, Ben-Menachem T, Chandrasekhara V, Chathadi K, Decker GA, et al. Guidelines for endoscopy in pregnant and lactating women. Gastrointest Endosc. 2012;76(1):18–24.
12. Sharma VK, Nguyen CC, Crowell MD, Lieberman DA, de Garmo P, Fleischer DE. A national study of cardiopulmonary unplanned events after GI endoscopy. Gastrointest Endosc. 2007;66(1):27–34.
13. Wexner SD, Beck DE, Baron TH, Fanelli RD, Hyman N, Shen B, et al. A consensus document on bowel preparation before colonoscopy: prepared by a task force from the American Society of Colon and Rectal Surgeons (ASCRS), the American Society for Gastrointestinal Endoscopy (ASGE), and the Society of American Gastrointestinal and Endoscopic Surgeons (SAGES). Gastrointest Endosc. 2006;63(7):894–909.
14. Wu KL, Rayner CK, Chuah SK, Chiu KW, Lu CC, Chiu YC. Impact of low-residue diet on bowel preparation for colonoscopy. Dis Colon Rectum. 2011;54(1):107–12.
15. Lim YJ, Hong SJ. What is the best strategy for successful bowel preparation under special conditions? World J Gastroenterol. 2014;20(11):2741–5.
16. Soweid AM, Kobeissy AA, Jamali FR, El-Tarchichi M, Skoury A, Abdul-Baki H, et al. A randomized single-blind trial of standard diet versus fiber-free diet with polyethylene glycol electrolyte solution for colonoscopy preparation. Endoscopy. 2010;42(8):633–8.
17. DiPalma JA, Brady CE III. Colon cleansing for diagnostic and surgical procedures: polyethylene glycol-electrolyte lavage solution. Am J Gastroenterol. 1989;84(9):1008–16.
18. Park S, Lim YJ. Adjuncts to colonic cleansing before colonoscopy. World J Gastroenterol. 2014;20(11):2735–40.
19. Pontone S, Angelini R, Standoli M, Patrizi G, Culasso F, Pontone P, et al. Low-volume plus ascorbic acid vs high-volume plus simethicone bowel preparation before colonoscopy. World J Gastroenterol. 2011;17(42):4689–95.
20. Corporaal S, Kleibeuker JH, Koornstra JJ. Low-volume PEG plus ascorbic acid versus high-volume PEG as bowel preparation for colonoscopy. Scand J Gastroenterol. 2010;45(11):1380–6.
21. Pang KS, Durk MR. Physiologically-based pharmacokinetic modeling for absorption, transport, metabolism and excretion. J Pharmacokinet Pharmacodyn. 2010;37(6):591–615.
22. Hookey LC, Depew WT, Vanner SJ. Combined low volume polyethylene glycol solution plus stimulant laxatives versus standard volume polyethylene glycol solution: a prospective, randomized study of colon cleansing before colonoscopy. Can J Gastroenterol. 2006;20(2):101–5.
23. Adams WJ, Meagher AP, Lubowski DZ, King DW. Bisacodyl reduces the volume of polyethylene glycol solution required for bowel preparation. Dis Colon Rectum. 1994;37(3):229–33, discussion 33–34
24. Kilgore TW, Abdinoor AA, Szary NM, Schowengerdt SW, Yust JB, Choudhary A, et al. Bowel preparation with split-dose polyethylene glycol before colonoscopy: a meta-analysis of randomized controlled trials. Gastrointest Endosc. 2011;73(6):1240–5.
25. Eun CS, Han DS, Hyun YS, Bae JH, Park HS, Kim TY, et al. The timing of bowel preparation is more important than the timing of colonoscopy in determining the quality of bowel cleansing. Dig Dis Sci. 2011;56(2):539–44.
26. Longcroft-Wheaton G, Bhandari P. Same-day bowel cleansing regimen is superior to a split-dose regimen over 2 days for afternoon colonoscopy: results from a large prospective series. J Clin Gastroenterol. 2012;46(1):57–61.
27. Jafri SM, Monkemuller K, Lukens FJ. Endoscopy in the elderly: a review of the efficacy and safety of colonoscopy, esophagogastroduodenoscopy, and endoscopic retrograde cholangiopancreatography. J Clin Gastroenterol. 2010;44(3):161–6.
28. Connor A, Tolan D, Hughes S, Carr N, Tomson C. Consensus guidelines for the safe prescription and administration of oral bowel-cleansing agents. Gut. 2012;61(11):1525–32.
29. Saito K, Inamori M, Sekino Y, Akimoto K, Suzuki K, Tomimoto A, et al. Management of acute lower intestinal bleeding: what bowel preparation should be required for urgent colonoscopy? Hepato-Gastroenterology. 2009;56(94–95):1331–4.
30. Chan WK, Saravanan A, Manikam J, Goh KL, Mahadeva S. Appointment waiting times and education level influence the quality of bowel preparation in adult patients undergoing colonoscopy. BMC Gastroenterol. 2011;11:86.
31. Abuksis G, Mor M, Segal N, Shemesh I, Morad I, Plaut S, et al. A patient education program is cost-effective for preventing failure of endoscopic procedures in a gastroenterology department. Am J Gastroenterol. 2001;96(6):1786–90.

32. Shaikh AA, Hussain SM, Rahn S, Desilets DJ. Effect of an educational pamphlet on colon cancer screening: a randomized, prospective trial. Eur J Gastroenterol Hepatol. 2010;22(4):444–9.
33. Spiegel BM, Talley J, Shekelle P, Agarwal N, Snyder B, Bolus R, et al. Development and validation of a novel patient educational booklet to enhance colonoscopy preparation. Am J Gastroenterol. 2011;106(5):875–83.
34. Tae JW, Lee JC, Hong SJ, Han JP, Lee YH, Chung JH, et al. Impact of patient education with cartoon visual aids on the quality of bowel preparation for colonoscopy. Gastrointest Endosc. 2012;76(4):804–11.
35. Liu X, Luo H, Zhang L, Leung FW, Liu Z, Wang X, et al. Telephone-based re-education on the day before colonoscopy improves the quality of bowel preparation and the polyp detection rate: a prospective, colonoscopist-blinded, randomised, controlled study. Gut. 2014;63(1):125–30.
36. Kang JY, Ho KY. Different prevalences of reflux oesophagitis and hiatus hernia among dyspeptic patients in England and Singapore. Eur J Gastroenterol Hepatol. 1999;11(8):845–50.
37. Guidelines for credentialing and granting privileges for gastrointestinal endoscopy. American Society for Gastrointestinal Endoscopy. Gastrointest Endosc 1998;48(6):679–82.
38. Rodney WM, Weber JR, Swedberg JA, Gelb DM, Coleman WH, Hocutt JE Jr, et al. Esophagogastroduodenoscopy by family physicians phase II: a national multisite study of 2,500 procedures. Fam Pract Res J. 1993;13(2):121–31.
39. Guidelines for documentation in the gastrointestinal endoscopy setting. Society of Gastroenterology Nurses and Associates, Inc. Gastroenterol Nurs. 1999;22(2):69–97.
40. SGNA position statement on minimal registered nurse staffing for patient care in the gastrointestinal endoscopy unit. Gastroenterol Nurs. 2002;25(6):269–70.
41. Association of periOperative Registered Nurses. Recommended practices for managing the patient receiving moderate sedation/analgesia. AORN J. 2002;75(3):642–6. 9-52
42. Society of Gastroenterology Nurses and Associates. SGNA guidelines for nursing care of the patient receiving sedation and analgesia in the gastrointestinal endoscopy setting. Gastroenterol Nurs. 2000;23(3):125–9.
43. Sandlin D. Capnography for nonintubated patients: the wave of the future for routine monitoring of procedural sedation patients. J Perianesth Nurs. 2002;17(4):277–81.
44. Lazzaroni M, Bianchi PG. Preparation, premedication and surveillance. Endoscopy. 2003;35(2):103–11.
45. Morrow JB, Zuccaro G Jr, Conwell DL, Vargo JJ II, Dumot JA, Karafa M, et al. Sedation for colonoscopy using a single bolus is safe, effective, and efficient: a prospective, randomized, double-blind trial. Am J Gastroenterol. 2000;95(9):2242–7.
46. OSHA clarifies, updates Bloodborne Pathogens Standard. Rep Med Guidel Outcomes Res. 2000;11(18):9–10, 12.

2 Colonoscopic Polypectomy: Punch, Snaring and EMR

Dae Kyung Sohn

2.1 Introduction

All colorectal polyps detected by colonoscopic examination, should be removed immediately or biopsied for planning a treatment. Most of polyps can be treated with various polypectomy methods [1–3]. For choosing the appropriate technique, endoscopists have to consider the polyp size, the location and morphological characteristics. Endoscopic biopsy only should be carefully performed before deciding a treatment plan especially for flat lesions including laterally spreading tumors, because it can make a fibrotic scar change and cause a difficult polypectomy. In this chapter, I will discuss the important principles and tips of performing a successful polypectomy.

2.2 General Considerations

The polyp should be characterized prior to removal. Polyp size, shape and exact location should be noted, and clear photographic documentation is also mandatory. If its boundary is unclear, dye-spraying or submucosal injection of a saline-dye mixed solution can be helpful [4–9]. Common biopsy forceps have jaws with 2.5 mm in diameter, which open to a width of 6–9 mm. Thus, photography of a polyp with opened jaws of the biopsy forceps can be helpful to estimate a polyp size objectively (Fig. 2.1).

For the successful polypectomy, it is also essential to make the optimized endoscopic views. All luminal residues should be removed by water flushing and suctioning, and then the lumen should be adequately distended. The targeted polyp should be located in the 5–6 o'clock position where polypectomy accessories emerge from the scope (Fig. 2.2). It is therefore usually helpful to

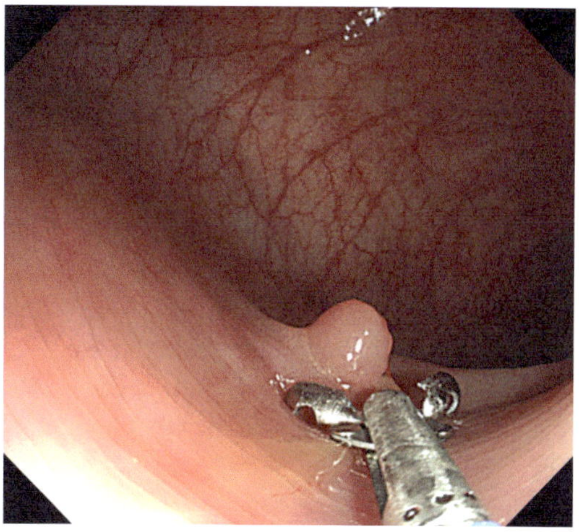

Fig. 2.1 Estimating polyp size using biopsy forceps. The biopsy forceps have jaws with 2.5 mm in diameter, which open to a width of 7 mm

D.K. Sohn, M.D., Ph.D.
National Cancer Center, Goyang-si, Gyeonggi-do, South Korea
e-mail: gsgsbal@ncc.re.kr

D.K. Sohn (ed.), *Practice and Principles in Therapeutic Colonoscopy*,
https://doi.org/10.1007/978-3-662-46552-3_2

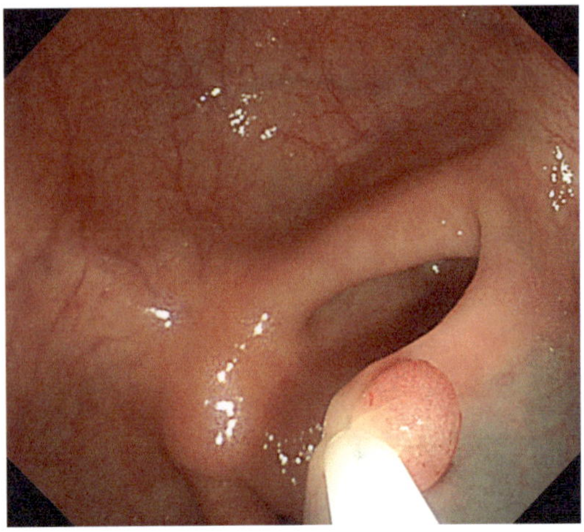

Fig. 2.2 The targeted polyp was located in the 5–6 o'clock position where polypectomy accessories emerge from the scope during polypectomy

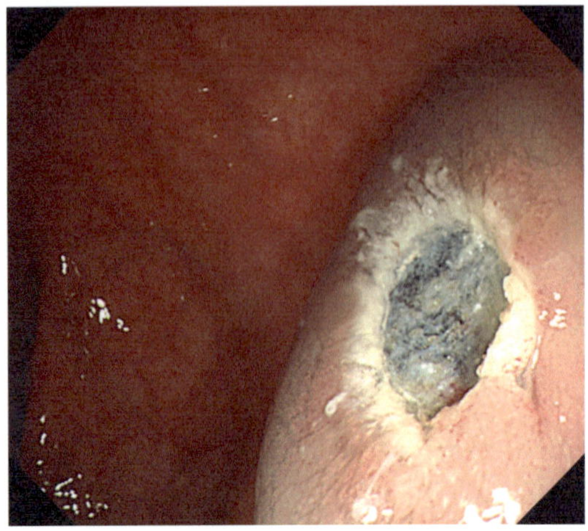

Fig. 2.3 Photographic documentation of tumor base should be recorded after polypectomy

rotate the scope or occasionally to change the patient's position. The endoscopist should be familiar with all endoscopic accessories and the diathermy unit. Especially, the power of the diathermy unit is recommended to be checked with regular intervals. The training of the assistant and the communication between the endoscopist and the assistant are also an essential for the safe procedures of polypectomy. Following resection, the endoscopist should carefully check the site to ensure all pathology has been clearly removed and to look for signs of bleeding or perforation. After polypectomy, photographic documentation is again needed (Fig. 2.3).

2.3 Indications and Contraindications

It is important to remember that most polyps identified at colonoscopy won't cause the patient harm immediately. In most cases the adenoma-carcinoma sequence progresses slowly. The endoscopist should therefore always consider the likely natural history of the lesion, the age and comorbidity of the patient and the risks of the intervention, prior to the procedure. However, the malignant potential of individual polyps is never known and even small, diminutive polyps can occasionally develop to cancers. It is therefore advisable that all polyps should be removed unless they are obviously non-neoplastic.

Polypectomy should not be attempted on a lesion that does not lift after submucosal saline injection (Fig. 2.4) [10–12]. Non-pedunculated polyps with overt signs of invasion are also best tattooed and biopsied (Fig. 2.5). Although some specialists are resecting large mucosal lesions or focal non-lifting tumor using endoscopic submucosal dissection techniques, the endoscopist should only consider removing lesions within their level of experience. Polyps found in close to colorectal cancers should be documented rather than removed since polypectomy

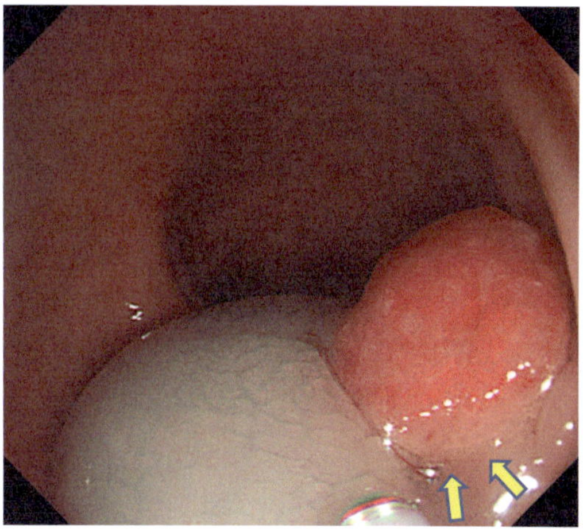

Fig. 2.4 Positive non-lifting sign

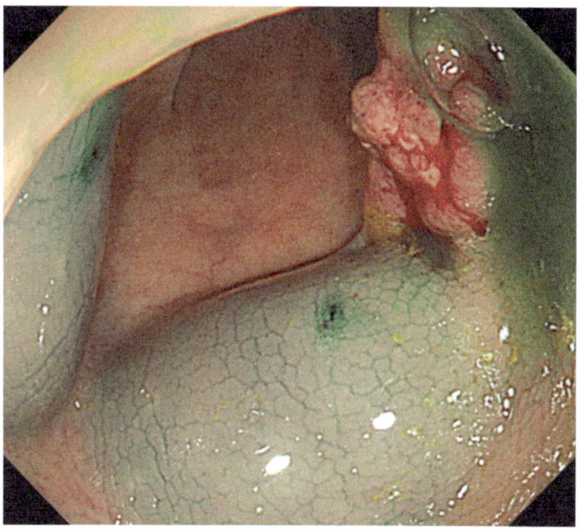

Fig. 2.5 Endoscopic tattooing for tumor localization before surgical resection

adds an unnecessary risk if the polyp lies within the resection margins of the tumor. Moreover, some endoscopists suggest that synchronous polyps with proximal colorectal cancers should be removed after appropriate surgical resection of the tumor, because tumor seeding may occur into recent polypectomy sites. Polypectomy should not be undertaken in patients with uncorrected bleeding disorders. Although aspirin and non-steroidal anti-inflammatory drugs do not appear to increase the risk following standard polypectomy, these agents are probably best discontinued for 1 week before planned removal of large or complex lesions. Platelet aggregation inhibitors are felt to pose a particular risk and are also best discontinued 1 week before polypectomy. Good bowel preparation is not only critical for polyp detection but reduces the risk of poor outcome including post-polypectomy syndrome or perforation. Loss of the resected polyp also can be occurred in this situation. Thus, re-scheduling the procedure should be recommended when the endoscopist finds a polyp in the presence of poor bowel preparation.

2.4 Specific Polypectomy Techniques

2.4.1 Cold Biopsy

A cold biopsy technique is useful for removal of diminutive polyps and avoids the risks associated with thermal injury. The open jaws should be targeted carefully to efficiently remove all abnormal tissue (Fig. 2.6). Large cup biopsies are helpful occasionally. Although this technique is very easy and safe, it has several disadvantages. First, it has a chance to leave residual tissue. Second, it is inefficient when polyp size is over the size of the cup of the forcep jaws. Thirdly, the endoscopic field may become obscured with blood with subsequent biopsies necessitating flushing. The technique is probably best reserved for the smallest of polyps.

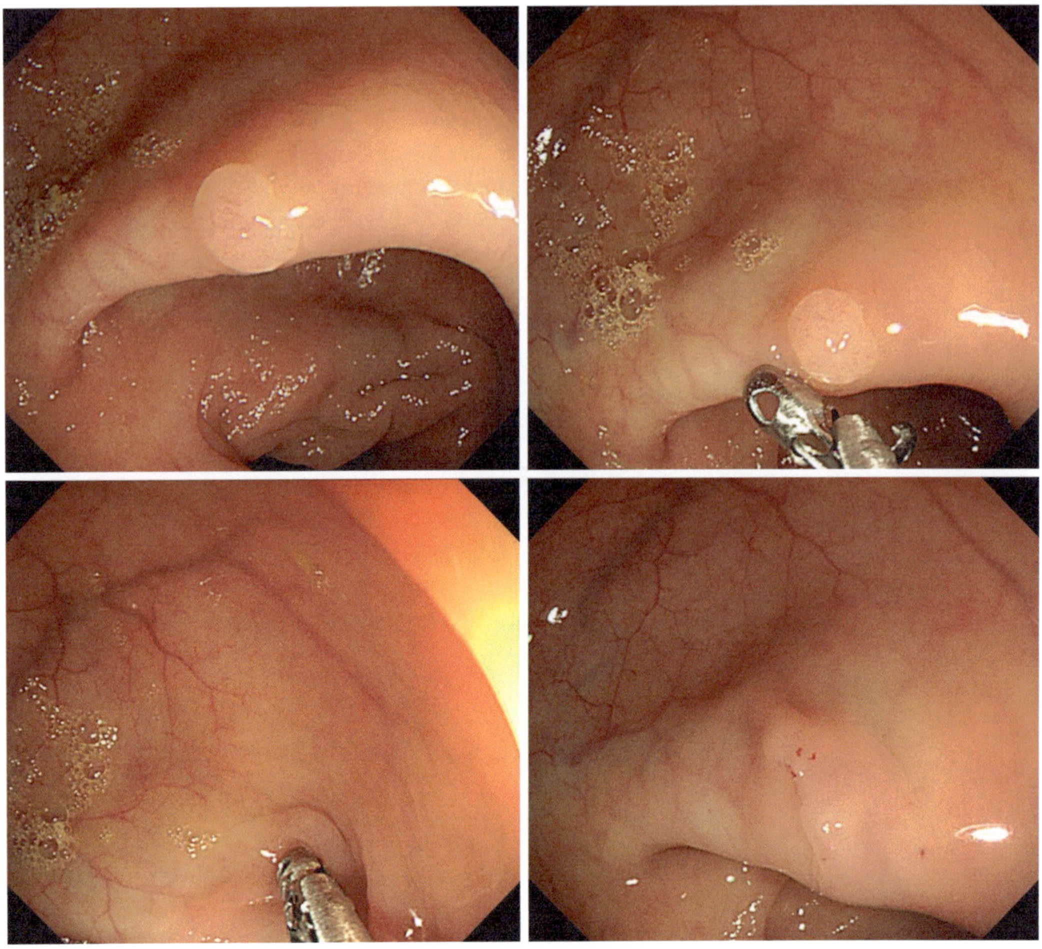

Fig. 2.6 Cold biopsy procedure

2.4.2 Hot Biopsy

Hot biopsy is an alternative technique for removing diminutive polyps. It uses both the mechanical force and the electrical burn to remove the abnormal tissue. Because of the risks of transmural thermal injury, it is best avoided in the right colon where the colonic wall is thin. It is now less commonly used than before, because there are a few reports showing that the risk of postpolypectomy bleeding may be increased after hot biopsy. During the procedure, the tip of the polyp is grasped and then tented away from the wall to create a pseudo stalk. Electrocautery is then applied and, since current density concentrates at the narrowest point, the pseudo stalk is cauterized and the tip is then avulsed for histological analysis. The endoscopist should watch carefully during electrocoagulation to avoid the excessive spread of thermal injury to the bowel wall (Fig. 2.7).

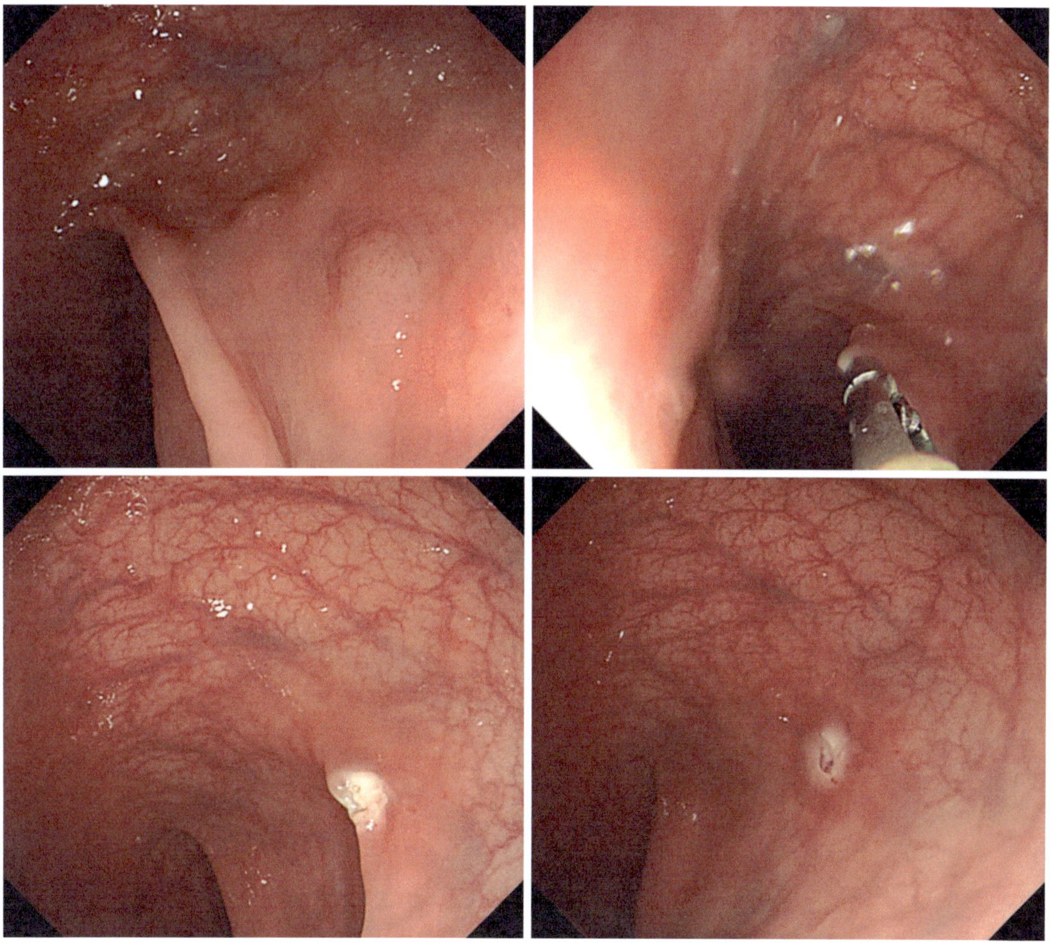

Fig. 2.7 Hot biopsy procedure

2.4.3 Cold Snaring

Cold snaring is a useful technique which is safe and effective in removing polyps up to 7 mm in diameter. It is more effective than biopsy at completely removing polyp tissue. Smaller snares are generally easier to manipulate over diminutive and small polyps. Some recommend also taking a 1–2 mm rim of normal tissue when undertaking cold snaring, if possible. Deflating the colonic lumen, to reduce wall tension, sometimes helps the polyp enter into the polypectomy snare. Once the snare has been closed, the polyp should be moved around to ensure only the mucosal surface (Fig. 2.8).

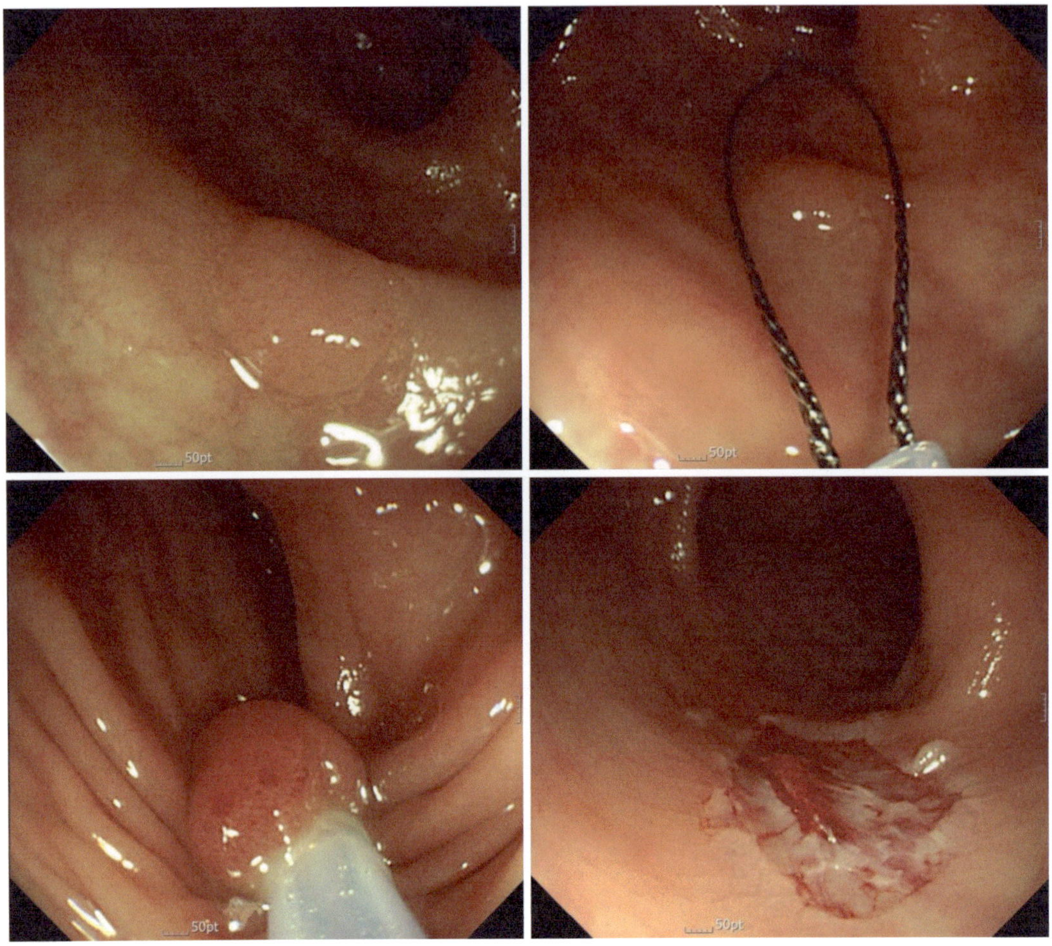

Fig. 2.8 Cold snaring procedure

2.4.4 Hot Snaring

The technique of hot snare polypectomy is similar to that of cold snaring up to the point of snare closure. During hot snaring, both mechanical and electrical forces are simultaneously acting to the polyp base (Fig. 2.9). This technique is most widely used for pedunculated and semi-pedunculated type polyps. Tenting of the ensnared polyp is recommended prior to the application of electrocautery to lift the point of diathermy away from the muscle layer and to minimize the risk of transmural injury (Fig. 2.9). For the safe snaring procedures, it is important to assistant's skill of controlling the snare. Some endoscopists prefer to operate the snare handle themselves during the application of cautery current to avoid the problems relating to communication with an assistant. Most experts recommend low power coagulation (25 W) for both hot biopsy and snare polypectomy, but both blended current and the more recently introduced Endocut system can be reasonably employed. Snare closure is a more important determinant of tissue heating than both time and power setting. The endoscopist should therefore exert firm squeeze pressure during the application of the cautery current.

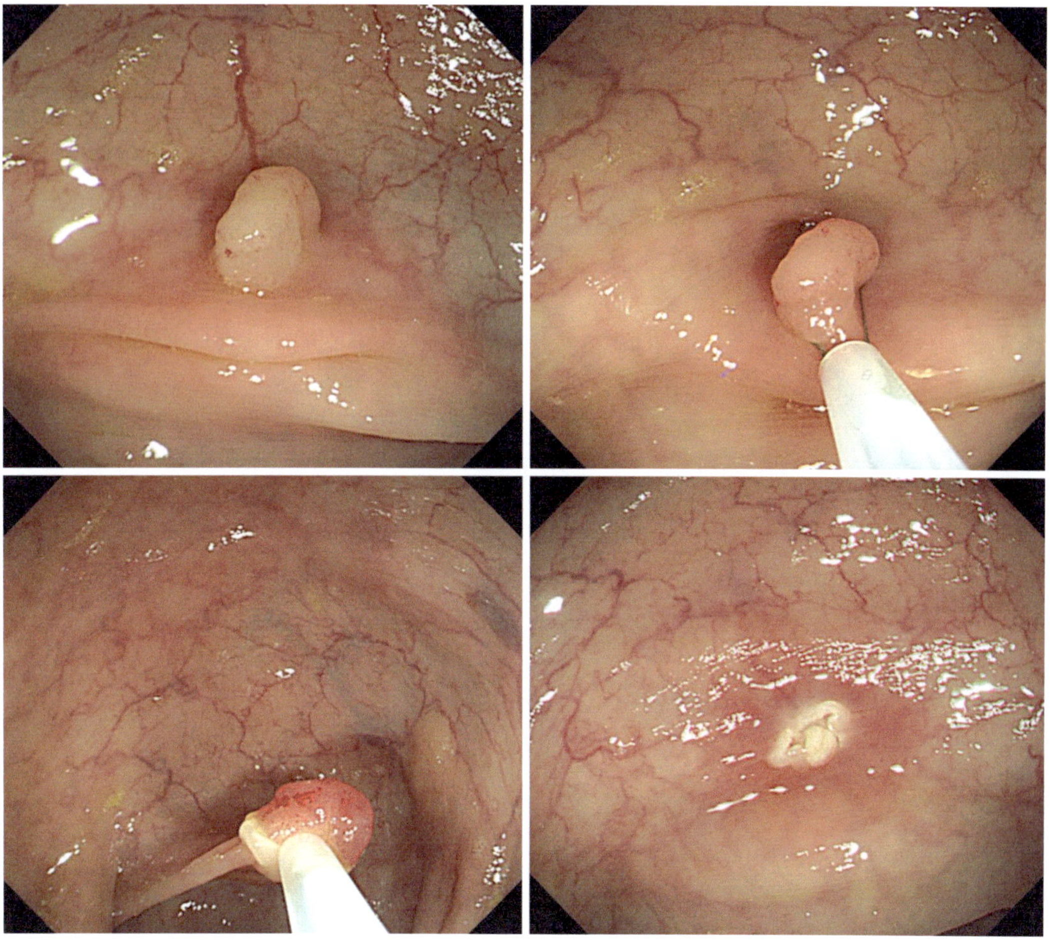

Fig. 2.9 Snaring polypectomy

2.4.5 Endoscopic Mucosal Resection

Submucosal injection beneath a flat or sessile mucosal lesion lifts it away from the muscle layer. This technique has several potential benefits. Firstly, lifting the lesion away from the muscle layer reduces the risk of transmural thermal injury as the point of polypectomy is moved away from the muscle layer. Secondly, it raises a flat lesion onto a sessile dome which is more readily ensnared. Finally, it identifies lesions invading or tethered to the deep submucosa or muscle layer (the non-lifting sign) which are unlikely to be suitable for endoscopic removal [10–12]. Many endoscopists use saline with or without adrenaline but a wide variety of solutions are available and may result in longer lasting cushions. For performing EMR, the endoscopist should clearly identify the margins of the lesion in order to avoid incomplete resection. Add of indigo carmine to the injection solution may help and some recommend marking the periphery of the lesion with electrocautery spots, and it can be beneficial to identifying the pit pattern of the lesion. A first injection just proximal to the margin of the lesion is often advantageous as the resulting dome tilts the lesion towards the endoscope making it easier to snare (Fig. 2.10). As the needle passes into the loose areolar connective tissue of the submucosa, the saline rapidly expands the space producing the characteristic dome. The endoscopist should be liberal with the injection volume, ensuring adequate separation between the lesion and the muscle layer (Fig. 2.11). Submucosal injection can also help to get the safe margin for resecting pedunculated

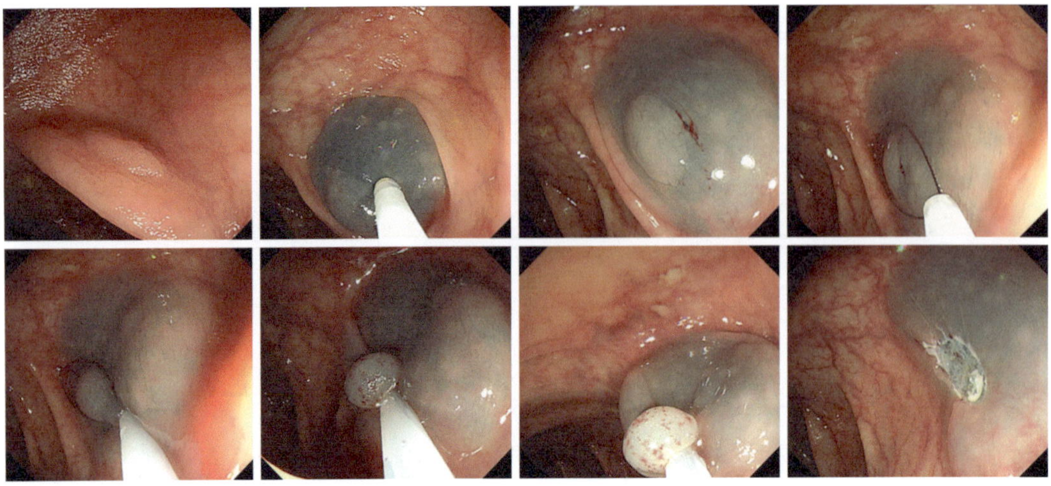

Fig. 2.10 Endoscopic mucosal resection procedure

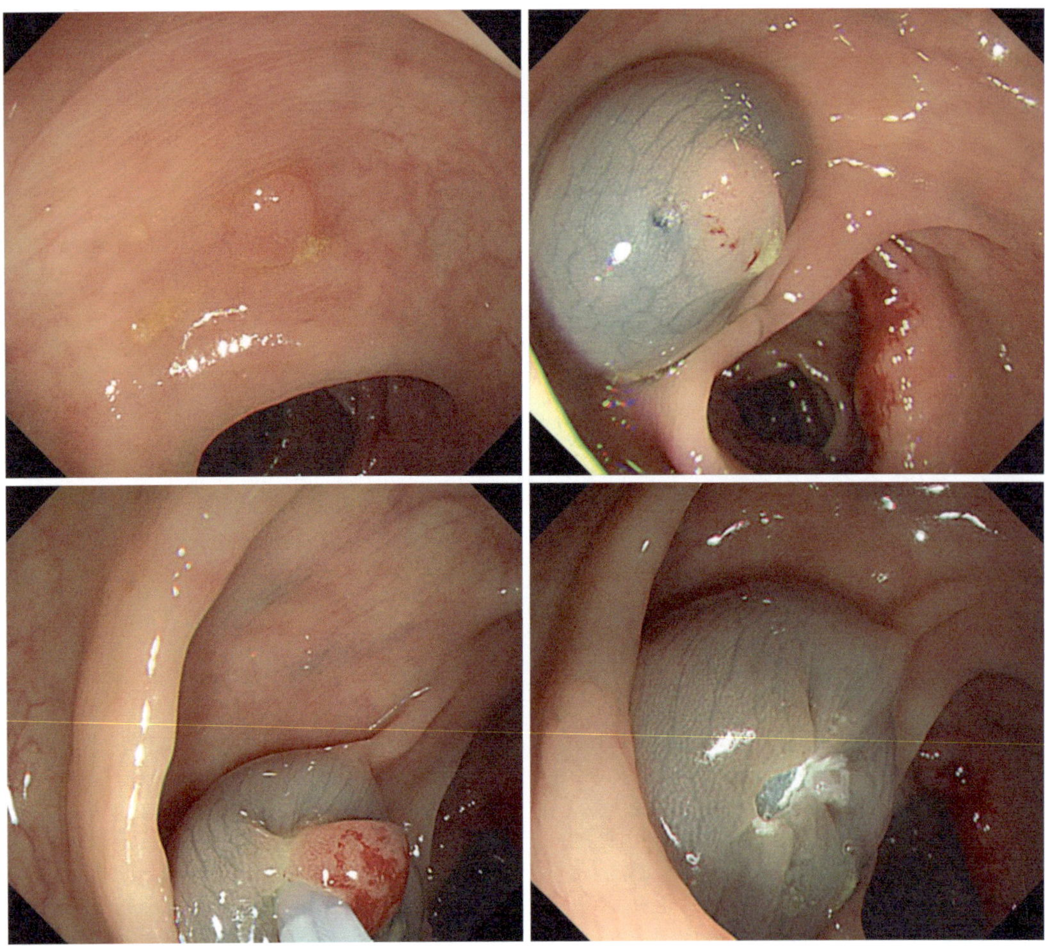

Fig. 2.11 Endoscopic mucosal resection: adequate separation between the lesion and the muscle layer

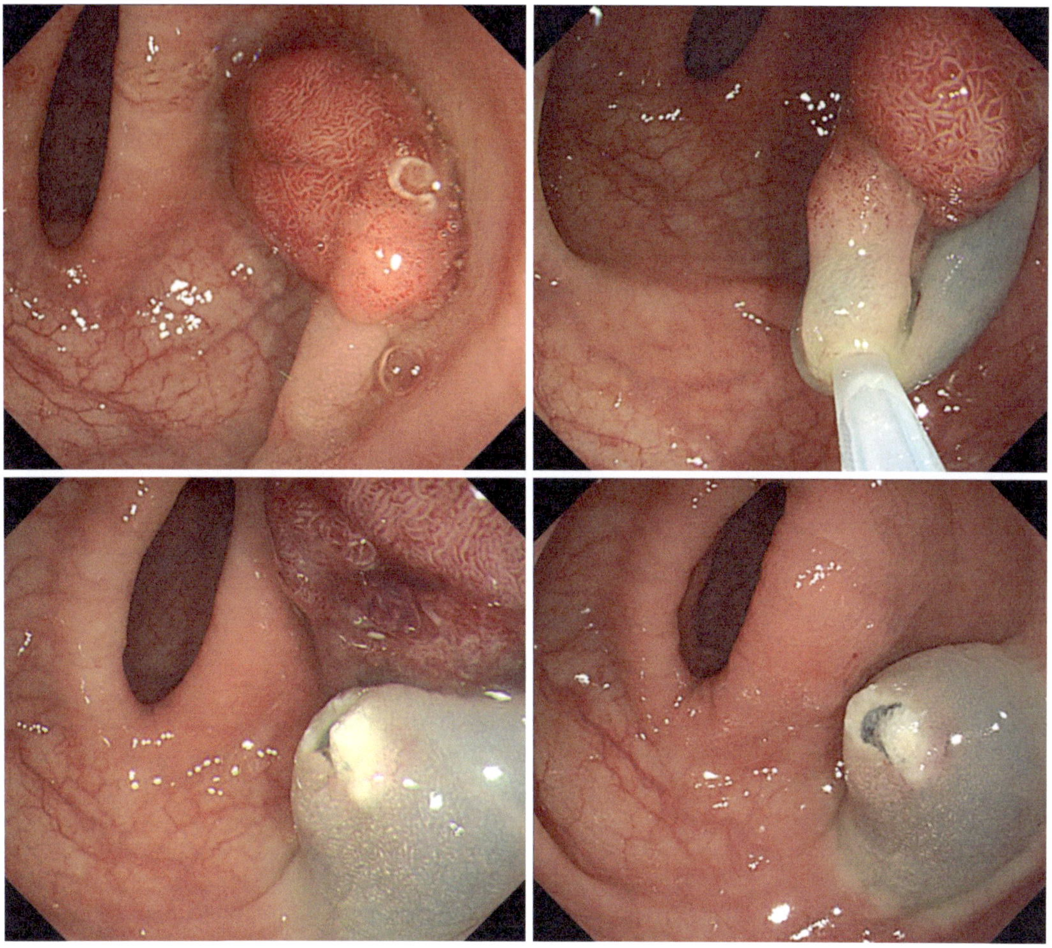

Fig. 2.12 Injection is helpful for safe cutting a pedunculated polyp

polyps (Fig. 2.12). A barbed or toothed snare may be helpful for gaining additional purchase on the resulting dome. Reducing wall tension by aspirating air also helps to draw the lesion into the loop of the snare. Some recommend taking a rim of normal tissue with the lesion. The entrapped lesion should be moved to ensure the muscle layer has not been snared and then diathermy applied in the usual way. Cap-assisted techniques or detachable loop snares are available but are used only in special circumstances (Fig. 2.13).

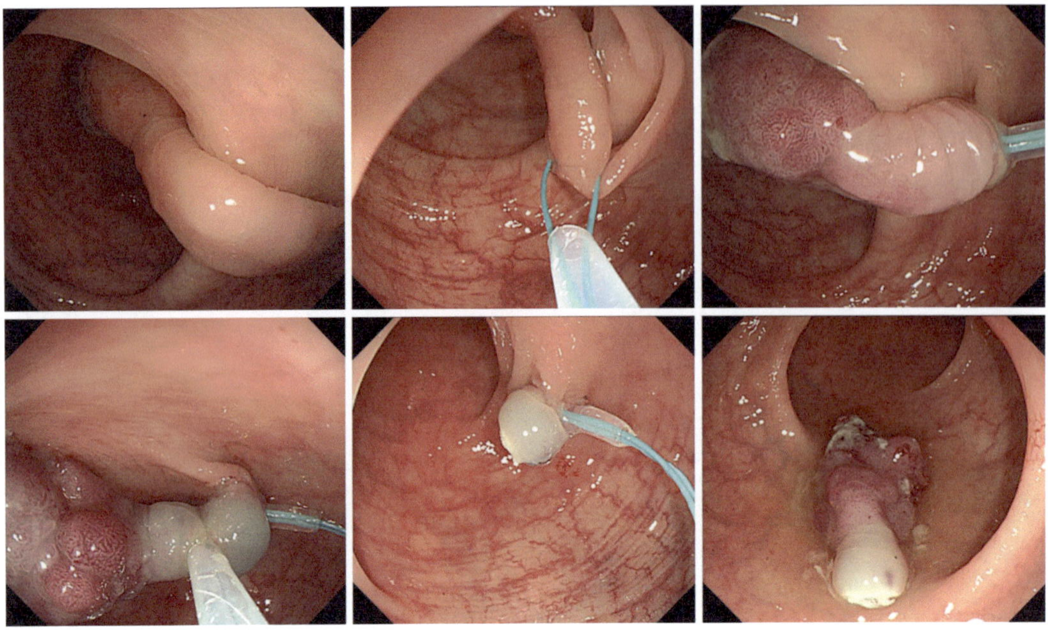

Fig. 2.13 Endoscopic mucosal resection using a detachable loop snare for removing a polyp with large stalk

2.5 Choosing the Polypectomy Techniques

For choosing the appropriate polypectomy technique, endoscopists have to consider the polyp size, shape, location and operability of the scope. Diminutive polyps less than 5 mm in diameter can be removed by cold biopsy regardless of polyp shape and location. Hot biopsy also can be used for removal of diminutive polyp up to 5 mm, especially in the left colon. However, the endoscopist must be careful to use it in the right colon due to the risks of postpolypectomy bleeding or postpolypectomy syndrome.

Cold snaring is a useful technique for removing sessile polyps up to 7 mm in diameter. Pedunculated polyps can be safely removed by hot snare polypectomy. However, EMR techniques after submucosal injection are recommended for removal of larger sessile polyps (more than 7 mm) and the pedunculated polyp with thick stalk. Flat and depressed lesions should be removed by EMR. Endoscopists should confirm that the depressed lesion is well lifted after submucosal injection, because it has a high risk of submucosal invasion.

Ideally, all polyps should be removed clearly without fragmentation. However, piecemeal resection can be used for flat or sessile lesions >2 cm. Recently, endoscopic submucosal dissection is also recommended for the en-bloc resection of large sessile polyps or laterally spreading tumors.

References

1. Karita M, Tada M, Okita K, Kodama T. Endoscopic therapy for early colon cancer: the strip biopsy resection technique. Gastrointest Endosc. 1991;37(2):128–32.
2. Karita M, Tada M, Okita K. The successive strip biopsy partial resection technique for large early gastric and colon cancers. Gastrointest Endosc. 1992;38(2):174–8.
3. Karita M, Cantero D, Okita K. Endoscopic diagnosis and resection treatment for flat adenoma with severe dysplasia. Am J Gastroenterol. 1993;88(9):1421–3.
4. Tsuga K, Haruma K, Fujimura J, Hata J, Tani H, Tanaka S, et al. Evaluation of the colorectal wall in normal subjects and patients with ulcerative colitis using an ultrasonic catheter probe. Gastrointest Endosc. 1998;48(5):477–84.
5. Shirai M, Nakamura T, Matsuura A, Ito Y, Kobayashi S. Safer colonoscopic polypectomy with local submucosal injection of hypertonic saline-epinephrine solution. Am J Gastroenterol. 1994;89(3):334–8.

6. Yamamoto H, Koiwai H, Yube T, Isoda N, Sato Y, Sekine Y, et al. A successful single-step endoscopic resection of a 40 millimeter flat-elevated tumor in the rectum: endoscopic mucosal resection using sodium hyaluronate. Gastrointest Endosc. 1999;50(5):701–4.
7. Waye JD, Lewis BS, Yessayan S. Colonoscopy: a prospective report of complications. J Clin Gastroenterol. 1992;15(4):347–51.
8. Kanamori T, Itoh M, Yokoyama Y, Tsuchida K. Injection-incision-assisted snare resection of large sessile colorectal polyps. Gastrointest Endosc. 1996;43(3):189–95.
9. Waye JD. Saline injection colonoscopic polypectomy. Am J Gastroenterol. 1994;89(3):305–6.
10. Uno Y, Munakata A. The non-lifting sign of invasive colon cancer. Gastrointest Endosc. 1994;40(4):485–9.
11. Ishiguro A, Uno Y, Ishiguro Y, Munakata A, Morita T. Correlation of lifting versus non-lifting and microscopic depth of invasion in early colorectal cancer. Gastrointest Endosc. 1999;50(3):329–33.
12. Han KS, Sohn DK, Choi DH, Hong CW, Chang HJ, Lim SB, et al. Prolongation of the period between biopsy and EMR can influence the nonlifting sign in endoscopically resectable colorectal cancers. Gastrointest Endosc. 2008;67(1):97–102.

3 Management of Large Sessile Polyps: EPMR vs. ESD

Eui-Gon Youk

3.1 Laterally Spreading Tumor

Development of the endoscopic techniques has had a major contribution to the diagnosis of early pathologic lesions. Now a day, the role of endoscopy is not only diagnostic tools but also treatment modality. In addition, as colonoscopy is enforced widely as a colorectal cancer screening test, the advanced polyps and early colorectal cancer is increased. It means that needs for the therapeutic endoscope is also increasing.

Most colorectal polyps are protruded or pedunculated type. It can be removed by snare polypectomy easily. About 7–36% of colorectal tumors are flat or depressed lesions which are known to have a high possibility of submucosal invasion comparing to pedunculated polyps [1–3]. These sessile or non-polypoid colorectal polyps are still challenging to remove endoscopically.

The laterally spreading tumor (LST) is a colorectal neoplasm, larger than 10 mm in diameter, characterized by a horizontally extending growth pattern with a relatively low vertical axis. LSTs are classified into two types, the granular (LST-G) and non-granular (LST-NG) types depending on the presence or absence of a surface nodularity. The granular type consists of collecting nodules that form uneven granular or nodular surfaces, whereas the non-granular type exhibits a flat, smooth surface. The detection of the LST-NGs is also not easy. To avoid missing these lesions, we should take note of pale redness, little deformation of wrinkles, loss of blood vessels.

The LST-G is subclassified into homogeneous (G-H) and nodular mixed (G-NM) types and the LST-NG into flat elevated (NG-FE) and pseudo-depressed (NG-PD) types. LSTs have been regarded as less invasive than other polypoid tumors of similar size. However it is important to observe the lesion carefully before deciding the treatment, because LSTs have different malignant potentials depending on its type. Nodular mixed tumors were associated more frequently with a villous adenoma component, and the giant nodules or concavities present in nodular mixed tumors were related to malignant potential. The LST-NGs, especially pseudo-depressed types, have a higher malignant potential than LST-Gs [4] and thus are considered a good indication for ESD to avoid unintended piecemeal resections (Fig. 3.1).

The size and type of LSTs are good predictors of invasive cancer, and the proportion of submucosal carcinoma increases with increasing size of flat depressed types. Non-granular LSTs larger than 30 mm were submucosal invasive carcinoma in 60% of cases. In contrast, homogeneous tumors are not associated with submucosal invasive carcinoma, even when they are larger than 30 mm.

E.-G. Youk, M.D., Ph.D.
Daehang Hospital, Seoul, South Korea
e-mail: youkgon@hanmail.net

D.K. Sohn (ed.), *Practice and Principles in Therapeutic Colonoscopy*,
https://doi.org/10.1007/978-3-662-46552-3_3

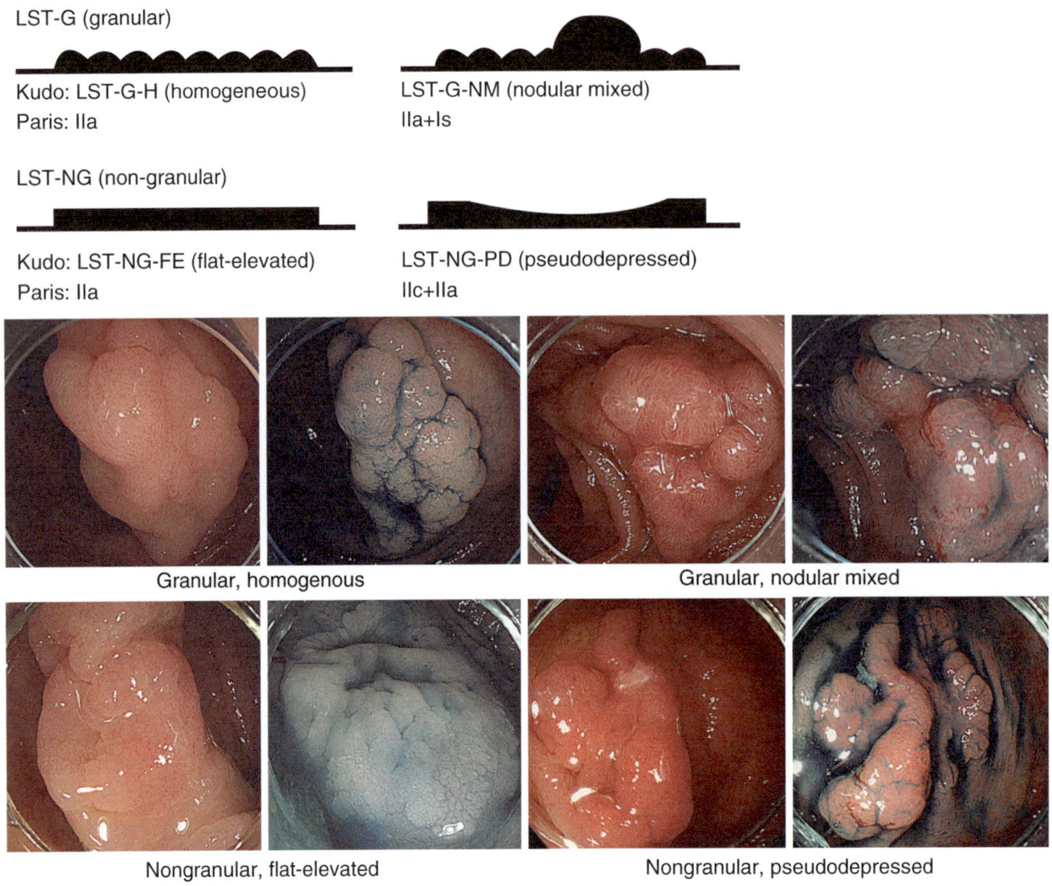

Fig. 3.1 Classification of LSTs

Generally, large size, depressed phenotype, and large nodules (≥10 mm) are known to be predictive markers of invasive carcinoma in LSTs [5].

In treating LSTs, conventional endoscopic mucosal resection (EMR) or endoscopic piecemeal resection (EPMR) technique can be suitable for homogeneous tumors. It is also recommended that flat elevated or pseudo-depressed or nodular mixed tumors larger than 20 mm, should be managed using endoscopic submucosal dissection (ESD) with en-bloc resection by the experienced endoscopists.

3.2 EPMR vs. ESD

EMR can replace the surgery in the treatment of early colon cancer without lymph node metastasis. Most colorectal polyps can be treated using simple snaring or EMR, although large sessile colorectal tumors exceeding 20 mm can't be removed by traditional EMR procedure. For these tumors, piecemeal resection is recommended [6]. The merit of piecemeal resection is that it is safe for resecting large sessile polyp. LSTs with granular homogenous type can be safely treated by EPMR, even it is larger than 30 mm. However, the fragmentation of specimens during conventional polypectomy or EMR prevents the evaluation of the resection margin involvement or the depth of tumor invasion, making it difficult to plan further treatment. In addition, any tumor cells remaining after piecemeal polypectomy can grow on the polypectomy scar and invade the submucosal layer more rapidly. Thus care should be used to remove suspicious malignant tumor including pseudo-depressed type LSTs by EPMR [6–8]. ESD introduced to overcome these limitations is now widely used for excising various gastrointestinal tumors, including colorectal tumors. ESD results in higher rates of en-bloc tumor resection, reducing local recurrences and providing more accurate pathologic information for planning further treatment. However, the procedure time is much longer and the complication rate is much higher for ESD than for EMR, limiting the use of ESD in the removal of colorectal tumors [9, 10].

According to several studies reported the outcomes of ESD, en-bloc resection rate is 84.9% (95% CI, 77.8–90.8), curative resection rate is 75.4% (95% CI, 66.7–82.2). A study on the long term outcomes of colorectal ESD found that the local recurrence rate was 2%, and the 3 and 5 year disease free survival rates were 97% and 95%, respectively. Safety outcomes of colorectal ESD are also important, in as much as perforation associated with this procedure was reported in 3.3–20.4%, with tumor size and the presence of fibrosis being independent risk factors for perforation [11–14]. Although many cases showing perforation have been improved with conservative treatment without surgery, using endoscopic clipping, it make to prolonged hospitalization and to need additional treatments.

In summary, both EPMR and ESD techniques can be used for large sessile polyps or LSTs. EPMR technique has merits of safety, ease and demerits of the difficulty of pathologic evaluation, high rates of local recurrences. ESD technique has merits of en-bloc resection, low rate of recurrence and demerits of long operation time, high rates of complications. Thus, ESD should be recommended for LSTs with suspected malignancy or lesions are technically difficult to treat with conventional EMR, and EPMR should be recommended for adenomatous lesions, LSTs with granular homogenous type [12, 15–18].

3.3 Indication of ESD

Basically, all endoscopic treatment is recommended only for lesions diagnosed as non-invasive tumors with a low metastatic potential. The risk factors for lymph node metastasis are poorly differentiated, signet-ring cell, and mucinous adenocarcinoma, massive submucosal invasion, lymphovascular invasion and tumor budding.

Table 3.1 Indications for ESD for colorectal tumors[a]

Lesions for which endoscopic en bloc resection is required
1. Lesions for which en bloc resection with snare EMR is difficult to apply
LST-NG, particularly LST-NG (PD)
Lesions showing a VI-type pit pattern
Carcinoma with shallow T1 (SM) invasion
Large depressed-type tumors
Large protruded-type lesions suspected to be carcinoma[b]
2. Mucosal tumors with submucosal fibrosis[c]
3. Sporadic localized tumors in conditions of chronic inflammation such as ulcerative colitis
4. Local residual or recurrent early carcinomas after endoscopic resection

[a]Partially modified from the draft proposed by the Colorectal ESD Standardization Implementation Working Group

[b]Including LST-G, nodular mixed type

[c]As a result of a previous biopsy or prolapse caused by peristalsis of the intestine

Current indications for colorectal ESD include (1) early colorectal cancer, (2) laterally spreading tumors ≥2 cm in diameter, (3) submucosal tumors, and (4) colorectal polyps with fibrosis. In detail, ESD study group in Japan announced the indication of colorectal ESD include LSTs with non-granular pseudo-depressed type, mucosal lesions with fibrosis caused by inflammation or scar change after biopsy, the tumor with underlying ulcerative colitis, recurred tumors after EMR resection, etc. They excluded the size criteria, more than 20 mm, in ESD indication, because depressed-type tumors with less than 20 mm in size can invade submucosal layer. And they also commented the submucosal infiltration of tumors should be shallow (Table 3.1).

3.4 Preoperative Diagnosis

Before procedure, malignant potential and margins should be clearly identified. Tumor morphology including color, unevenness, depression, fold convergence also carefully evaluated. Malignant tumors have the loss of the surface pattern of pits or the structure of micro-vessels. Dye spraying, magnifying endoscopy, narrow band image can be helpful to identifying it. For predicting the malignant polyps, the accuracy of conventional endoscopy is about 80%, and that of chromo-magnifying endoscopy is up to 96–98%. Endoscopic ultrasonography (EUS) is also helpful to diagnose the submucosal invasive cancer, however it is still not popular because the additional equipment is required.

3.5 ESD Instruments

3.5.1 Knifes

Some kinds of knifes are used for ESD treatment of colon tumors. The Dual knife (Olympus Optical Co., Tokyo, Japan) is most commonly used, and also the Flush knife BT (Fujifilm Medical, Tokyo, Japan) and the Jet B-knife (ZeonMedical, Tokyo, Japan) which are capable of injecting the submucosa solution, are used for colorectal ESD. A notable characteristic of the Jet B-knife is the use of the bipolar current system—it can minimize the damage to the muscle layer and reduce the risk of perforation. The Insulated tip knife-nano (IT-nano, Olympus Optical Co.) has also been developed and have been utilized in colorectal ESD, which has a merit of bringing out the relatively fast treatment. The Hook knife (Olympus Optical Co.) can be used to lift and cut the tissues in cases of the LSTs with fibrosis or the difficult-to-reach tumors. And recently, the clutch cutter (Fujifilm Corp., Tokyo, Japan) of grasping-type scissor forceps and the SB knife Jr. (Sumitomo Bakelite Co., Tokyo, Japan) has been developed and used (Fig. 3.2).

3.5.2 Hemostatic Forceps

The Hemostat-Y (H-S2518; Pentax) of a bipolar-type hemostatic Forceps and the Coagrasper (FD-410LR; Olympus Medical Systems Co., Tokyo, Japan) of a monopolar-type forceps have been currently used in ESD procedures.

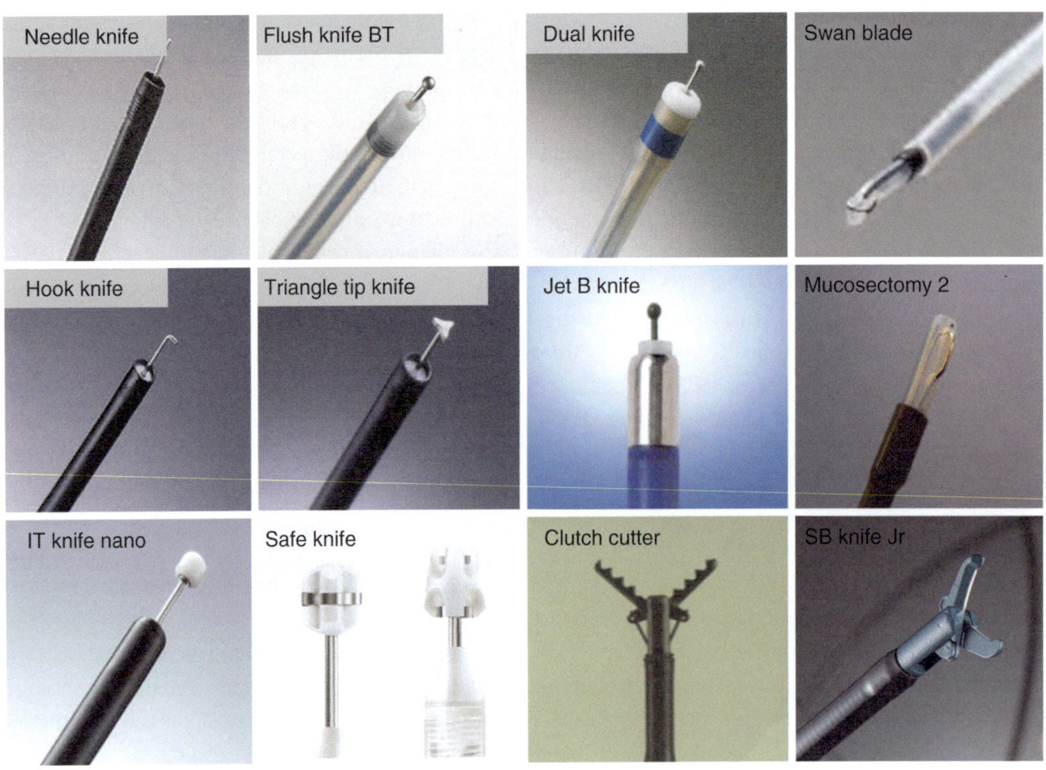

Fig. 3.2 Various endoscopic knives

3.5.3 Distal Attachments

Various distal attachments such as a standard transparent cap or the ST hood short-type (DH-28GR and 29CR; Fujifilm Medical Co., Tokyo, Japan) are useful for colorectal ESD. A transparent cap is usually attached at the distal end of the endoscope, which make it easy to dissect the submucosal layer with lifting up the lesions. This also can be used as an auxiliary tool for compressing the tissue during bleeding (Fig. 3.3).

3.5.4 Submucosal Injection Solutions

The maintenance of the sufficient submucosal elevation using injecting hypertonic solutions is essential for the success of the ESD. An ideal submucosal injection solution should be inexpensive, readily available, non-toxic, easy to prepare and inject, and should provide a long-lasting submucosal cushion. The normal saline solution is the most commonly used as the injection solution for conventional EMR. Saline-epinephrine injection has been shown to be an effective method for the complete endoscopic polypectomy, especially in flat or sessile lesions. However, other substances such as sodium hyaluronate, hydroxypropyl methylcellulose and glycerol, have been preferred for ESD procedures because of their ability to create a longer lasting submucosal cushion as a result of their viscous properties. A small amount of Indigo Carmine is also mixed to the submucosal-injecting solution to enhance the lesion and margins. Recently the ready-to-use sodium hyaluronate also commercially available—MucoUp® (Seikagaku Co., Tokyo, Japan) and Endo-ease (Unimed Co., Seoul, Korea).

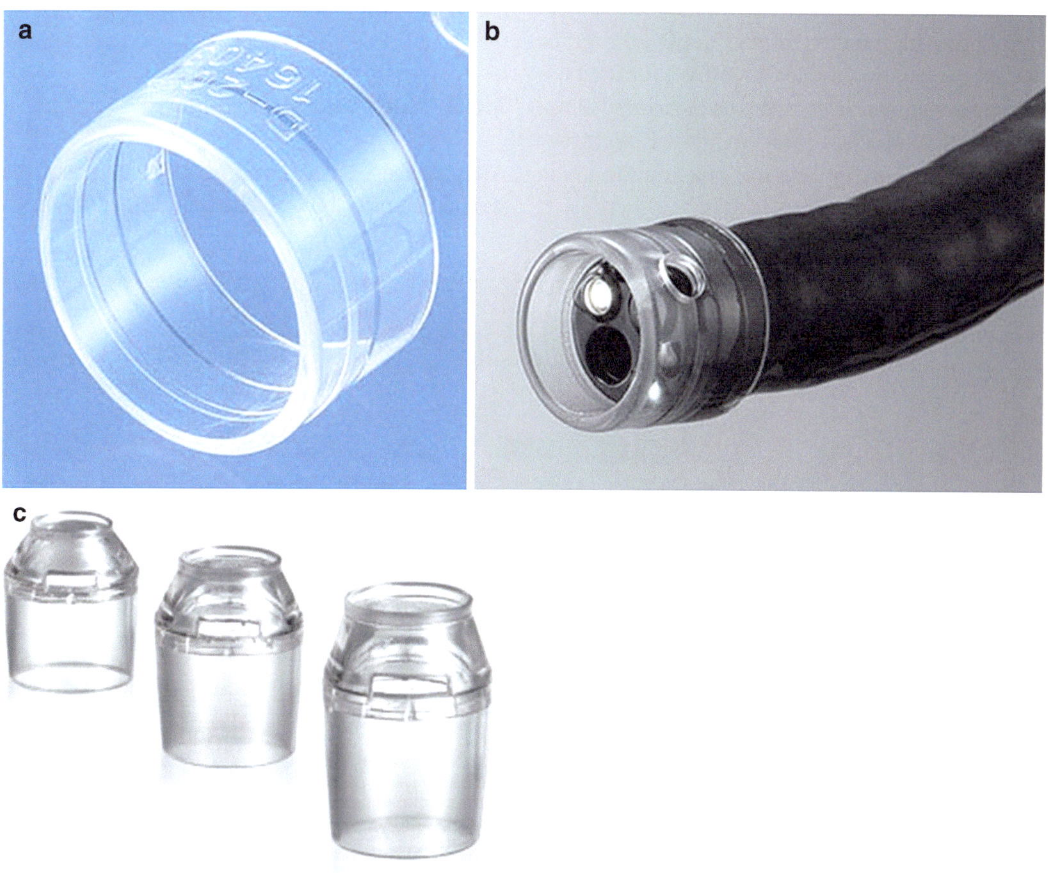

Fig. 3.3 (**a**) A transparent hood (D 201-16403; Olympus, Tokyo). (**b**) The tip of the colonoscope attached to the transparent hood. (**c**) Small-caliber transparent (ST) hood

3.5.5 CO_2 Insufflation Systems

The use of carbon dioxide (CO_2) gas is usually recommended in colorectal ESD. The CO_2 insufflation into the colonic lumen has been proven effective to let the patient stand the long ESD procedure and to reduce the risk of pneumoperitoneum in cases of perforation and other complications. Operators should pay always attention to abdominal distension due to over-insufflation of the gas during ESD procedures.

3.5.6 Electrosurgical Generators

For ESD procedures, the multi-functioning electrosurgical generators are usually used, such as the VIO300D (ERBE, Tübingen, Germany) or the ESG100 (Olympus Medical Co.). The ERBE generator was set to the Endo-Cut mode (Effect 3, 60–80 W) for incision of the mucosa, and to the Endo-Cut mode (Effect 3, 60–80 W) or forced coagulation mode (40–50 W) for incision of the submucosa. Bleeding was controlled using hemostatic forceps, such as the Coagrasper (Olympus Optical) in the soft coagulation mode (50–80 W).

3.6 ESD Procedures

3.6.1 Incision of Mucosa

Because the boundary of colon lesions is usually clear, mucosal marking is non-essential for colorectal ESD. Only marking is needed for selective cases with a blurred margin. Generally, mucosal incision was made around margin with at least 5 mm after submucosal injection. For lifting flap easily, an initial mucosal incision was recommended in more than 1 cm apart from margin. And it is not recommended that the 360° surrounding incision around a tumor have been made without enough submucosal dissection because the leak of the injection solutions from the submucosal layer leads the loss of fields of views in submucosal layers and make it difficult to complete dissection. In order to achieve the complete dissection, it is necessary to formulate the strategy including the repeated sequences of submucosal injection, mucosal incision and submucosal dissection (Fig. 3.4).

3.6.2 Submucosal Dissection

After making initial mucosal incision, firstly we should attempt the submucosal dissection up to

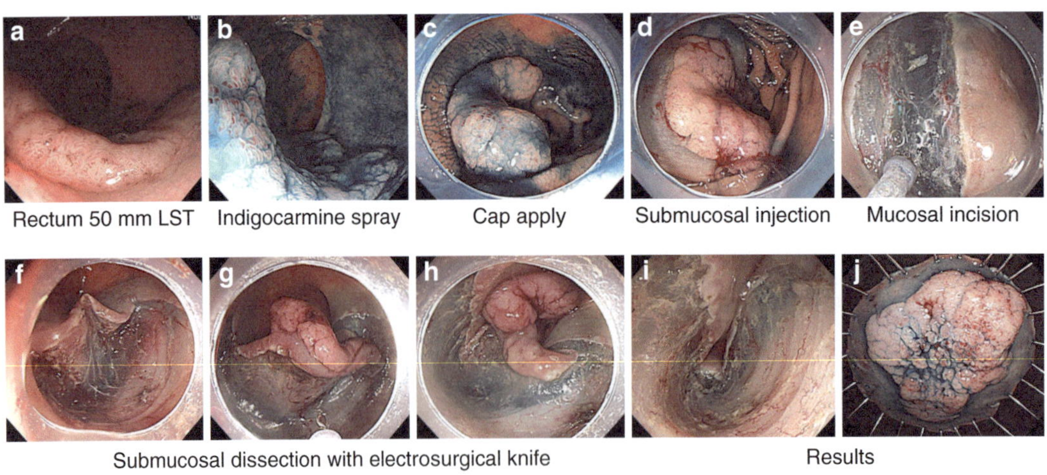

Fig. 3.4 ESD procedures. Endoscopic submucosal dissection for rectal neoplasia. (**a**) 50 mm sized middle rectal lesion which is a type 0-IIa, laterally spreading, intramucosal adenocarcinoma in adenoma. (**b**) Chromoendoscopic view with indigocarmine, showing demarcation of the margin of the lesion. (**c**) Cap applied. (**d**) Submucosal injection at the oral margin of the lesion, with the endoscope in a retroflexed position. (**e**) Initial mucosal incision at the anal margin of the lesion. (**f**) Extension of the incision in a circumferential manner around the lesion, with endoscope in a straight position. (**g**) Repetition of submucosal injections from the exposed submucosal layer. (**h**) Repetition of dissection of the submucosal connective tissue. (**i**) The artificial ulcer after removal. The vessels on the ulcer base are treated with hemostatic forceps to prevent bleeding. (**j**) Complete resection of the lesion in one piece

identifying the muscle layer. A cap or a hood of the tip of endoscopy could be helpful to lift the mucosal flap. After identifying the muscle layer, then submucosal dissection would be kept continuously going at the level of lower 1/3 of submucosal layers. When the vessels are met, it can be controlled by coagulation using a knife or a coagrasper. Small-sized vessels were managed by slow-moving of a knife with a swift mode or a forced coagulation mode. Large-sized vessels are needed to a coagulation by the coagrasper with a soft coagulation mode with 50–80 W.

For dissecting the areas with submucosal fibrosis or infiltration by tumor, a careful approach should be needed with identifying an exact plane of dissection. The ESD is limited in these situations, because it makes it easier to occur the perforation (Fig. 3.4).

3.7 ESD for Special Situations

A lots of problems during ESD can be occurred in the cases of difficult locations of tumors, in which endoscopy is not reach to the tumor base, rather than in cases with large-sized tumors. In general, the difficulty of ESD is growing as tumor locations from the rectum up to cecum. To dissect it easier during submucosal dissection, the endoscopy should be placed in parallel to the muscle layer. However, it is difficult to make it in cecum, angulated areas of colon including hepatic flexure, splenic flexure, etc. Sometimes, the retroflexion of the scope would be helpful for reaching to the tumor. And also patients' position change and air suction could be helpful (Fig. 3.5).

3.7.1 Rectal Lesions

ESD for rectal lesions is known to be easy, but ESD for the lesion closed to dentate line or anal canal is difficult because of the limited spaces. A perpendicular approach can be made by retroflextion of the scope, then the procedure from oral side to anal side is possible. The local anesthesia is also needed to reduce the pain during the dissection of tumors closed to anal canal. In this situation, the surgical local excision can be more preferred than ESD.

3.7.2 Sigmoid or Descending Colon

Sigmoid colon is severely bent and has the narrow interior space of the lumen. Because it is not

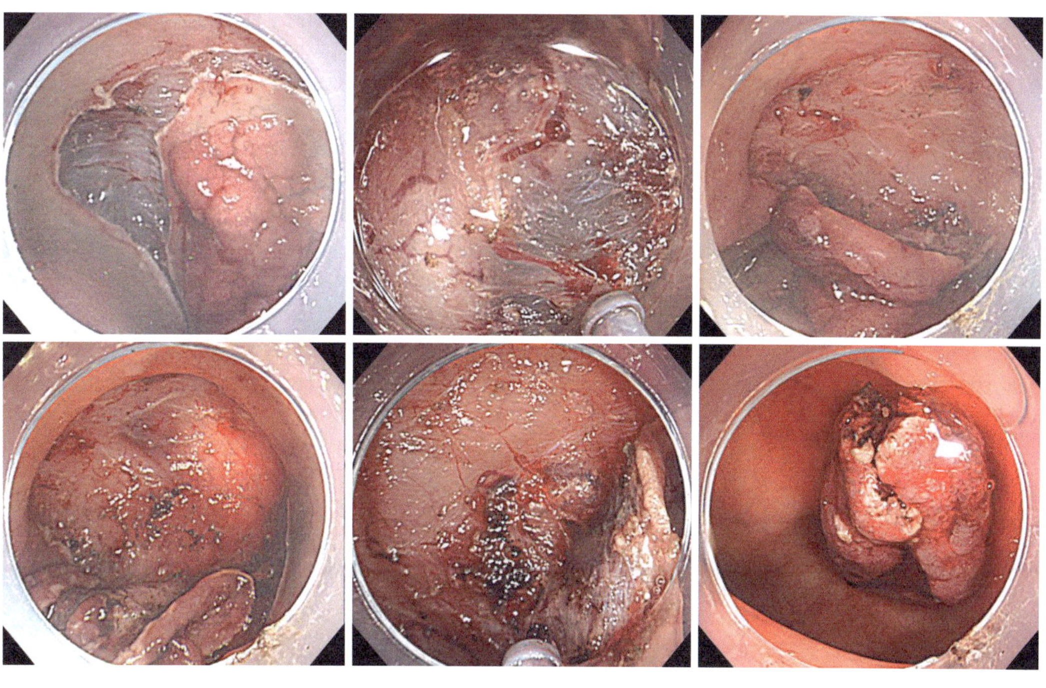

Fig. 3.5 Retroflexion method during submucosal dissection

attached to the retroperitoneum, it is freely movable and its shape can be altered during the procedure depending on the amount of air. Descending colon has also the narrow interior space of the lumen, even it is not much bent. It is difficult to perform ESD due to the limited movement of the scope. Because the endoscope is placed perpendicular to the lesion at the sigmoid-descending junction, it is hard to make a visualization of tumors. Endoscopists should not to try a retroflexion of the scope in sigmoid or descending colon. It is very a dangerous procedure because it is likely to damage a colon wall and to increase a risk of perforation.

3.7.3 Transverse Colon

The common problem of ESD at the transverse colon is a movement of colon due to an aortic pulsation and bowel peristalses. The patient's aortic pulsation may be exaggerated in a supine position. The change of patient's position such as the right decubitus or left decubitus can be helpful in this situation. However, the most important factor of deciding patients' position is that tumors must be placed at the opposite site to the gravity. It is very important to make a visualization of submucosal dissection plane. It is necessary to find an optimal position of the patient in every ESD procedures.

3.7.4 Hepatic Flexure Colon

The endoscopic blind spot can be made due to the curved folds and acute angulation of the hepatic flexure colon. It is also very difficult to perform ESD in hepatic flexure colon. If necessary, a hook-knife and an IT-knife can be helpful to lift and dissect the lesions which is placed perpendicular to the scope.

3.7.5 Cecum

It is very difficult to crossly approach to the dome-shape portion of the cecum. It is recommended to perform EMR or EPMR beside of ESD, if it looks like a benign lesion. However, if en-bloc resection is needed for a suspicious malignant lesion, various knives including a hook knife, a dual knife and an IT-nano knife would be used even time-consuming. The approaches from medial (ileocecal valve) to lateral (anti-mesenteric) would be helpful to complete ESD. Sometime it is needed to reduce the electrical power of the electro-surgical units for the safe dissection.

3.7.6 Appendiceal Orifice

It is better to enforce the surgical resection of cecum, if the tumor is in growing up into the appendiceal orifice. However, ESD can be tried when the tumor is located closely or focally involve to the appendiceal orifice. In this situation, the operator should explain to the patient in advance that acute appendicitis after EMR or ESD could be developed and that prophylactic antibiotics also could be needed.

3.7.7 Ileocecal Valve

Since the mucosal surface of the ileocecal valve is granular, it is easy to be overlooked even in the presence of adenomas. Sometimes the tumor located in the ileocecal valve can be grown up to the terminal ileum. Thus, it is not easy to perform ESD for tumors located at the ileocecal valve. However, the relatively-thickened wall of the ileocecal valve may reduce the chance of perforation during ESD. When the tumor is extended to the terminal ileum, it is better to dissect the ileal side firstly during ESD. The enough saline injection at the ileal submucosa can lead to the expulsion of the tumor from the ileum into the colon. Rapid dissection or excision of tumors can be performed at that time. Argon plasma coagulation is helpful for remove the remnant tumor at the terminal ileum. If the tumor involves the ileocecal valve circumferentially, it is very difficult to complete ESD. In this situation, the stricture can be occurred after complete removal of tumor by EPMR or ESD.

3.7.8 ESD in Submucosal Fibrosis

Submucosal fibrosis can be induced by cancer cell invasion, inflammation, etc. It is careful that the biopsy can make a submucosal fibrosis in flat tumors or the laterally spreading tumors. When there is severe submucosal fibrosis under the tumor, even a simple snaring is likely to make a perforation due to muscle injury. Thus, ESD is preferred to snaring or EMR in this situation. However, a non-lifting mucosal layer and a hard submucosal layer are not easy to make a visualization of a correct dissecting plane during ESD.

For setting the electrosurgical unit, a forced coagulation mode or a swift coagulation mode is commonly used during ESD. For the fibrotic lesions, it is helpful that the coagulation current is decreased and cutting current is increased.

The knife should be carefully moved to submucosal plane crossly in fibrotic areas. Because severe fibrosis can lead to an incorrect plane and to increase a muscle injury, the dissection of severe fibrotic areas could be recommended to leave it to the last minute during ESD. Although the mucosal lifting after saline injection is not enough at the fibrotic areas, the frequent submucosal injection is needed to visualize clearly a correct plane, even a little (Fig. 3.6).

3.8 Histopathology

For a precise histological diagnosis, which determines the need for additional treatment after ESD, a proper handling of resected specimens by ESD is required. Microscopic tissue diagnosis is performed through the series of processes including fixing the specimen in the plate, a formalin fixation, a gross observation and a section of the specimen.

3.8.1 Specimen Fixation and Histologic Diagnosis

The resected specimen by ESD is firstly fixed in a rubber or cork-sheet plate using several pins. And then it has to be fixed into the 10–20%

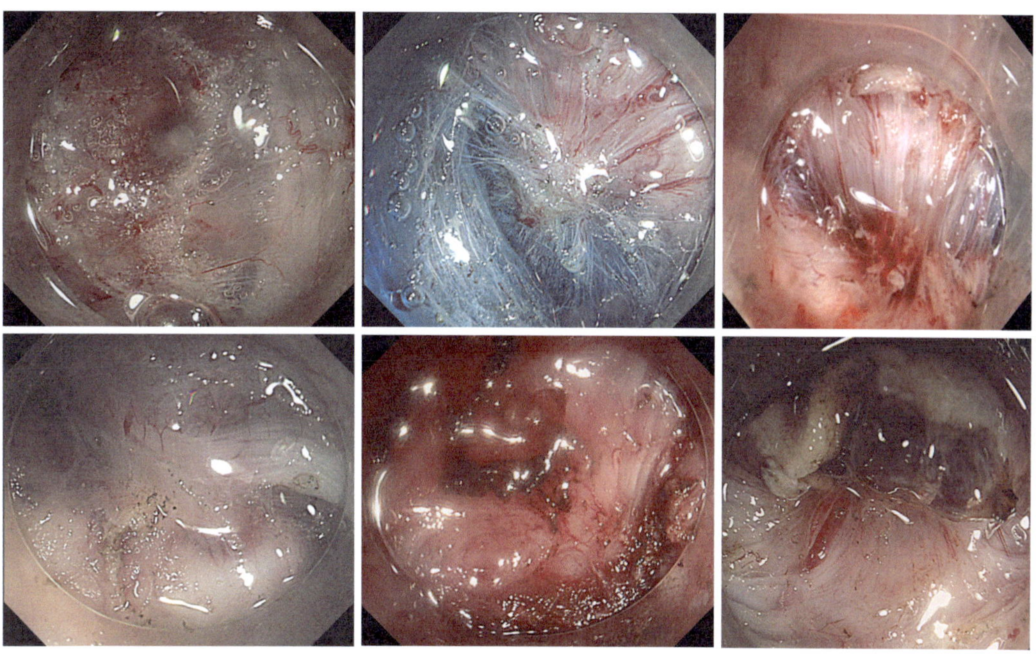

Fig. 3.6 Submucosal fibrosis. Non-lifting mucosal layer and a hard submucosal layer are not easy to make a visualization of a correct dissecting plane during ESD. *Upper three photos* were fibrosis without submucosal invasion and *lower three photos* were massive submucosal invasion or proper muscle invasion cases

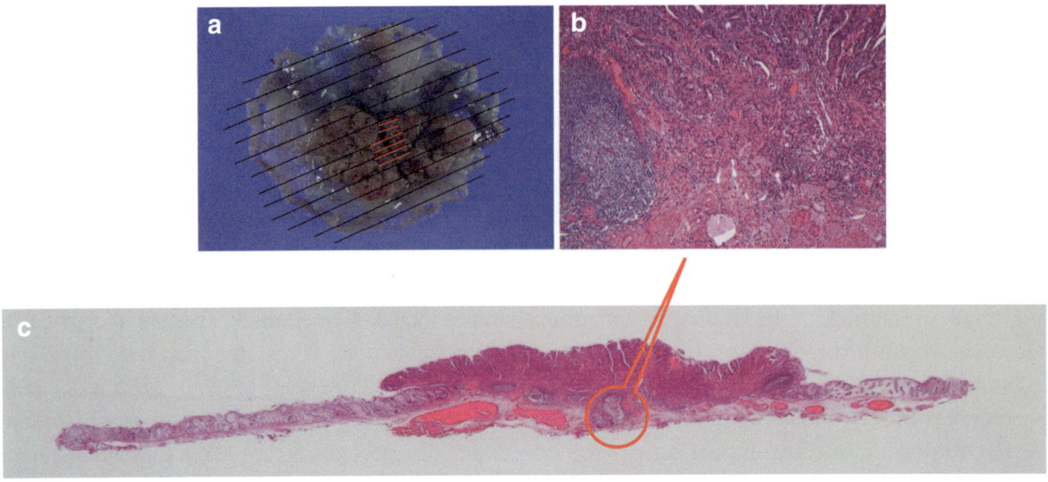

Fig. 3.7 Pathologic examination. (**a**) The specimen is fixed with formalin and sliced in 2- to 2.5-mm intervals. *Red lines* indicate the adenocarcinoma after mapping. (**b**) The adenocarcinoma is confined in the submucosa layer 500 μm sm1 depth with risk factor lymphovascular emboli (hematoxylin and eosin [H&E] stain, ×200). (**c**) Images arranged in line (H&E stain)

formalin solution after the saline-washing as soon as possible. The direction also should be marked in the specimen plate (Fig. 3.7).

A gross observation including the size, color, shape and hardness of the tumor is needed before cutting the tumor. It is important to decide the cutting line and sections through the discussion of clinical information and gross observation between the endoscopist and the pathologist.

Histologic diagnosis should be included to the histologic type, the depth of invasion, the presence of lymphovascular invasion, the resection margin including vertical and lateral, tumor buddings, a pattern of invasion. These factors are used for determining the additional treatment such as a radical surgery.

It would be necessary to surgical resection, if histopathology findings are shown to have one of follows; (1) deep submucosal invasion (sm2 or more), (2) if differentiation is bad (poorly differentiation), (3) mucinous carcinoma or signet-ring cell carcinoma, (4) lymphatic or vascular invasion, (5) positive tumor budding, (6) positive resection margin. Therefore, endoscopists should keep it in mind and try not to resect completely the tumor with deep submucosal invasion. And they also have to try to get an enough resection margin without tissue fragmentation.

Conclusions

When you perform the endoscopic treatment for colorectal lesions, you have to consider the indications, tumor location, size, depth of invasion, the skill of an endoscopist and the hospital facility for emergency surgery. Colorectal ESD is the most advanced skill in the fields of therapeutic endoscopy. Currently many of reports showed that ESD results in higher rates of en-bloc tumor resection, reducing local recurrences and providing more accurate pathologic information for planning further treatment. However, the procedure time is much longer and the complication rate much higher for ESD than for EMR. For the safe ESD procedures, endoscopists should be trained well to advance steadily.

References

1. Tsuda S, Veress B, Toth E, Fork FT. Flat and depressed colorectal tumours in a southern Swedish population: a prospective chromoendoscopic and histopathological study. Gut. 2002;51:550–5.
2. Saitoh Y, Waxman I, West AB, et al. Prevalence and distinctive biologic features of flat colorectal adenomas in a North American population. Gastroenterology. 2001;120:1657–65.

3. O'Brien MJ, Winawer SJ, Zauber AG, et al. Flat adenomas in the National Polyp Study: is there increased risk for high-grade dysplasia initially or during surveillance? Clin Gastroenter Hepatol. 2004;2:905–11.
4. Shin-ei K. Endoscopic treatment of neoplasms in colon and rectum. Tokyo: Igaku-Shoin Ltd.; 2000.
5. Tanaka S. Basic technique of endoscopic mucosal resection and endoscopic submucosal dissection for colorectal tumors – knack, pitfall, and conclusive evidence of adjustment. Japan: Medical View; 2006.
6. Soetikno RM, Gotoda T, Nakanishi Y, Soehendra N. Endoscopic mucosal resection. Gastrointest Endosc. 2003;57:567–79.
7. Pech O, May A, Gossner L, Rabenstein T, Ell C. Management of pre-malignant and malignant lesions by endoscopic resection. Best Pract Res Clin Gastroenterol. 2004;18:61–76.
8. Larghi A, Waxman I. State of the art on endoscopic mucosal resection and endoscopic submucosal dissection. Gastrointest Endosc Clin N Am. 2007;17:441–69.
9. Cao Y, Liao C, Tan A, Gao Y, Mo Z, Gao F. Meta-analysis of endoscopic submucosal dissection versus endoscopic mucosal resection for tumors of the gastrointestinal tract. Endoscopy. 2009;41:751–7.
10. Tanaka S, Oka S, Kaneko I, et al. Endoscopic submucosal dissection for colorectal neoplasia: possibility of standardization. Gastrointest Endosc. 2007;66:100–7.
11. Tanaka S, Terasaki M, Hayashi N, Oka S, Chayama K. Warning for unprincipled colorectal endoscopic submucosal dissection: accurate diagnosis and reasonable treatment strategy. Dig Endosc. 2013;25:107–16.
12. Saito Y, Fukuzawa M, Matsuda T, et al. Clinical outcome of endoscopic submucosal dissection versus endoscopic mucosal resection of large colorectal tumors as determined by curative resection. Surg Endosc. 2010;24:343–52.
13. Tanaka S, Haruma K, Oka S, et al. Clinicopathologic features and endoscopic treatment of superficially spreading colorectal neoplasms larger than 20 mm. Gastrointest Endosc. 2001;54:62–6.
14. Lee EJ, Lee JB, Lee SH, Youk EG. Endoscopic treatment of large colorectal tumors: comparison of endoscopic mucosal resection, endoscopic mucosal resection-precutting, and endoscopic submucosal dissection. Surg Endosc. 2012;26:2220–30.
15. Puli SR, Kakugawa Y, Saito Y, Antillon D, Gotoda T, Antillon MR. Successful complete cure en-bloc resection of large nonpedunculted colonic polyps by endoscopic submucosal dissection: a meta-analysis and systematic review. Ann Surg Oncol. 2009;38:493–7.
16. Fujishito M, Yahagi N, Nakamura M, et al. Endoscopic submucosal dissection for rectal epithelial neoplasia. Endoscopy. 2006;38:493–7.
17. Hurlstone DP, Atkinson R, Sanders DS, Thomson M, Cross SS, Brown S. Achieving R0 resection in the colorectum using endoscopic submucosal dissection. Br J Surg. 2007;94:1536–42.
18. Tanaka S, Kashida H, Saito Y, et al. JGES guidelines for colorectal endoscopic submucosal dissection/endoscopic mucosal resection. Dig Endosc. 2015;27:417–34.

Early Colorectal Cancer

4

Kyung Su Han

4.1 Introduction

Clinically, the name of "early cancer" suggests that the lesion is localized with potential for complete cure after resection. In 1963, the Japanese Research Society for Gastric Cancer defined "early gastric cancer (EGC)" as adenocarcinoma of the stomach confined to the mucosa or submucosa, irrespective of lymph node metastasis [1].

In the same with EGC, early colorectal cancer (ECC) is defined as a tumor that has not spread beyond the submucosal layer [2]. Thus, ECC includes cases of Tis (carcinoma in situ with intraepithelial involvement or invasion of the lamina propria) and T1 (tumor invades the submucosa).

On the base of TNM staging, Tis lesions make histopathologic distinction between stomach and the large bowel. While the Tis of the stomach include only carcinoma in situ (intraepithelial involvement), Tis of the large bowel include both carcinoma in situ and intramucosal carcinoma (invasion of the lamina propria). The reason why intramucosal carcinoma of the large bowel is regarded as Tis, is that there is no risk of lymph node metastasis in this lesion. By the same token, T1 lesion also make histopathologic distinction between stomach and the large bowel, as T1 of the stomach including intramucosal and submucosal lesion, and T1 of the large bowel include only the submucosal lesion.

In respect of pathologic classification of intramucosal neoplasia, there have been divergences of traditional terminology between Japan and Western countries, i.e., intramucosal carcinoma (Japan) and high-grade dysplasia (Western). But, around 2000, Asian, European, and American pathologists proposed the consensus, adopted in Vienna classification [3]. Later, the Vienna classification was revised in World Health Organization (WHO) classification of digestive tumors. According to the revised Vienna classification, both intramucosal carcinoma and high-grade dysplasia are classified as category 4 (mucosal high grade neoplasia) [4] (Table 4.1).

Recently, the incidence of ECC is increasing, and this may be possibly caused by that the number of people undergoing colonoscopic examination is growing. In terms of treatment, radical resection has been traditionally regarded as a standard therapy for ECC, like any other advanced colorectal cancer. However, with advances in instruments and techniques, endoscopic resection of ECC has developed. Moreover, in selective ECC cases, endoscopic resection is now accepted as a standard therapy. Thus, determining the endoscopic respectability has been a matter of operator's concern, and critical for planning the treatment strategy.

K.S. Han, M.D., Ph.D.
National Cancer Center, Goyang-si,
Gyeonggi-do, South Korea
e-mail: kshan@ncc.re.kr

D.K. Sohn (ed.), *Practice and Principles in Therapeutic Colonoscopy*,
https://doi.org/10.1007/978-3-662-46552-3_4

Table 4.1 The revised Vienna classification of gastrointestinal epithelial neoplasia

Category	Diagnosis
1	Negative for neoplasia
2	Indefinite for neoplasia
3	Mucosal low grade neoplasia
	Low grade adenoma
	Low grade dysplasia
4	Mucosal high grade neoplasia
4–1	High grade adenoma/dysplasia
4–2	Non-invasive carcinoma (carcinoma in situ)
4–3	Suspicious for invasive carcinoma
4–4	Intramucosal carcinoma
5	Submucosal invasion by carcinoma

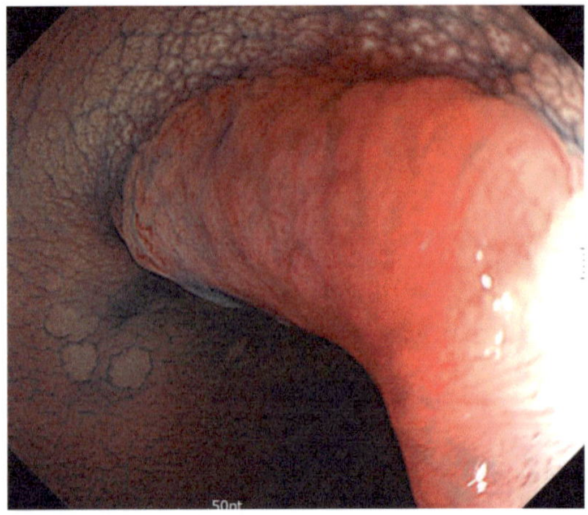

Fig. 4.1 Pit pattern type V & type I. Chromoendoscopic view of the polyp shows the PP type V (irregular or non-structured pattern), while circumferential mucosa shows the PP type I (round pattern)

4.2 Endoscopic Features Suggesting Malignancy

Usually, endoscopic findings are enough to distinguish colorectal benign lesions from malignant lesions. However, in some cases, endoscopic findings are so ambiguous that it is difficult to discriminate between benign and malignant. Although biopsy and pathologic examination are the only way to confirm the malignancy, the initial endoscopic evaluation may be of a great significance for planning the treatment strategy. Thus, endoscopist should be reminded on the endoscopic features strongly suggesting a malignant component.

According to data from US National Polyp Study, the size of polyp is strongly associated with malignancy potential. If the size of polyp is less than 5 mm in diameter, the prevalence of malignancy is less than 0.1%, that is, rarely malignant [5]. On the other hand, if a polyp is larger than 50 mm in diameter, the probability of malignancy is over 30% [6].

Malignant transformation is more frequent in villous type than in tubular type. And the other gross configurations suggesting malignant transformation are as follows; nodule on polyp ("Buddha-like" polyp), color change or easy-touch bleeding, depression or ulceration, firm consistency or induration, broadening of the stalk or fold irregularity, irregular surface contour and lack of air-induced deformation.

The orifices of colonic mucosal glands are called by pits, and the specific shape and arrangement of pits in each lesion is called by a pit pattern (PP). The pit pattern can be clearly observed with chromoendoscopy and it reflects the lesion's histological nature. Kudo et al. has firstly characterized pit patterns [7]. The pit patterns are classified into five types (I–V); PP type I (round pattern), PP type II (asteroid or papillary pattern), PP type III (tubular pattern), PP type IV (branch or gyrus-like pattern), PP type V (unstructured pattern). PP type III can be classified into two sub-types; PP type IIIs (small tubular pattern) and PP type IIIL (large tubular pattern). PP type V also can be classified into PP type Vi (irregular pattern) and PP type Vn (non-structured pattern). Among these PP types, PP type V carries very-high risks of malignant transformation (60–95%) [8] (Fig. 4.1).

Sano, et al. investigated the alterations of the surface capillary patterns, using a enhanced endoscopy called narrow band imaging (NBI) endoscopy [9]. It emphasize the superficial capillary structure without any dye, using the light of specific blue and green wavelengths. The colonic capillary patterns (CP) are classified into four patterns: CP type I (no meshed capillary vessels, faint pattern), CP type II (regularly meshed capillary vessel) and CP type III (irregularly meshed capillary vessels). CP type III lesions are divided into two sub-types, CP type IIIA (lack of uniformity, high density of capillary vessels) and CP type IIIB (loose capillary vessels or nearly avascular). Among these CP types, CP type III show very high incidence of malignant transformation (70–90%) [8].

4.3 Endoscopic Classification of Superficial Neoplastic Lesions

The concept of the "superficial neoplastic lesion" is very similar to that of early cancer. The superficial neoplastic lesion is the lesion with endoscopic features suggesting the limited invasion depth (no more than into the submucosa). The Japanese group classified the superficial neoplastic lesions as "type 0", distinguished from types of advanced lesions, i.e., the Borrmann type 1–4 [10, 11].

On 2002, an international group of endoscopist, surgeons, and pathologists participated in the Paris workshop, and explored the utility and clinical relevance of the Japanese endoscopic classification of superficial neoplastic lesions [12]. In the Paris workshop, the participants proposed a general framework for the endoscopic classification of the superficial neoplastic lesion (type 0). According to the Paris classification, type 0 lesion of large bowel is classified as three types basically, based on the absence or the presence of protrusion/ulceration. The basical three types include polypoid (type 0-I), non-polypoid, non-excavated (type 0-II), and non-polypoid, excavated (type 0-III) lesions (Fig. 4.2).

Type 0-I lesions are polypoid lesions, i.e., protruding type. With respect to the presence or the absence of neck, Type 0-I lesions are classified into two sub-types, pedunculated type (type 0-Ip) and sessile type (type 0-Is).

Type 0-II lesions are relatively flat lesions, neither protruded nor excavated. Type 0-II lesions are classified into three sub-types, slightly elevated type (type 0-IIa), flat type (type 0-IIb), and slightly depressed type (type 0-IIc). Among type 0-II lesions, some have both findings of elevation

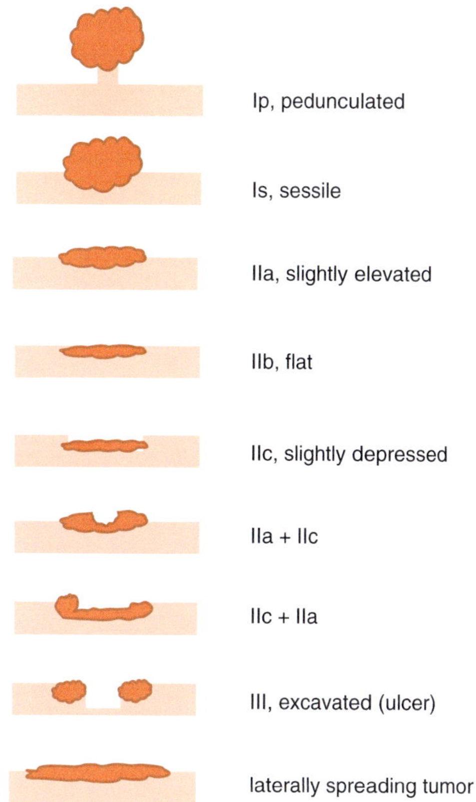

Fig. 4.2 Paris endoscopic classification of superficial neoplastic lesion

and depression. Type 0-IIc + IIa lesion is a depressed lesion with partially elevated area and type 0-IIa + IIc is an elevated lesion with partially depressed area.

Because both type 0-Is and 0-IIa lesions are all elevated type, sometimes it is difficult to make a distinction between type 0-Is and 0-IIa. The distinction between type 0-Is and type 0-IIa is based on the height of the lesion. When compared with the height of closed biopsy forceps (2.5 mm), type 0-Is lesions are >2.5 mm and type 0-IIa lesions are <2.5 mm. Type 0-III lesions are excavated lesions, i.e., ulcerated type.

Laterally spreading tumor (LST) is defined by lateral growth of lesions larger than 10 mm in diameter with a low vertical axis. Based on the surface morphology, LSTs are usually classified into two types, granular and non-granular type. The granular type LSTs are classified into two sub-types, the hemogenous type and the nodular mixed type. The non-granular type LSTs are classified into two sub-types, the flat elevated type and the pseudodepressed type [See Chap. 3]. Malignant transformation is more frequent in nodular mixed type and pseudodepressed type.

4.4 Endoscopic Resectability of Superficial Neoplastic Lesions

For planning the treatment strategy of the superficial neoplastic lesions (surgery or endoscopic resection), proper evaluation of endoscopic respectability is critical.

Although there are several unfavorable histopathological factors for lymph node metastasis in ECC, endoscopic respectability is absolutely depend on the invasion depth, because only the invasion depth is a predictable histopathologic factor before resection, and also it is technically difficult to completely resect the lesions with deep invasion.

Methods for evaluating the invasion depth of superficial neoplastic lesions include EUS, magnifying endoscopy, and the nonlifting sign.

EUS has a high level of accuracy for T staging, especially differentiation between Tis and T1 colorectal cancer (CRC), showing 90% accuracy in differentiation between Tis and T1 CRC [13, 14].

Magnifying chromoscopy is a reliable method for differentiating between non-neoplastic and neoplastic lesions, or between early cancer and adenoma [14, 15].

Clinically, in evaluation of invasion depth, making a differentiation between limited submucosal invasion and deep submucosal invasion is important. However, neither EUS nor magnifying endoscopy is suitable for making a differentiation between limited and deep submucosal invasion.

Checking for the nonlifting sign (NLS) is a simple and reliable method for making a differentiation between limited and deep submucosal invasion. NLS was first described by Uno et al. in 1994, defined as when the lesion is not lifted by saline solution injection into the submucosal layer of the tumor base [16] (Fig. 4.3). Lesions with deep submucosal invasion are not lifted by a submucosal saline solution injection because of the dense fibrosis associated with invasive carcinoma, which prevents fluid infiltration through the submucosal connective tissue. Some previous studies showed the correlations between deep submucosal invasion and the nonlifting sign. According to previous researches, ECC lesions with deep submucosal invasion show 72.7–100% of nonlifting sign, while lesions with limited submucosal invasions show 0–20% of nonlifting sign [17–19]. Although nonlifting sign is every effective for evaluating invasion depth, mechanical stimulation such as forceps biopsy may cause the false-positive event. Han, et al. reported that forceps biopsies may lead to submucosal fibrosis, causing the nonlifting sign in colorectal tumors although they have not invaded the deep submucosal layer. They also reported that an increase in the number of postbiopsy days (more than 21 days) may influence the nonlifting sign in endoscopically resectable colorectal tumors. They recommended that mechanical stimulation such as forceps biopsies should be minimized before endoscopic resection, and endoscopic resection should be tried as soon as possible if biopsy was performed [17].

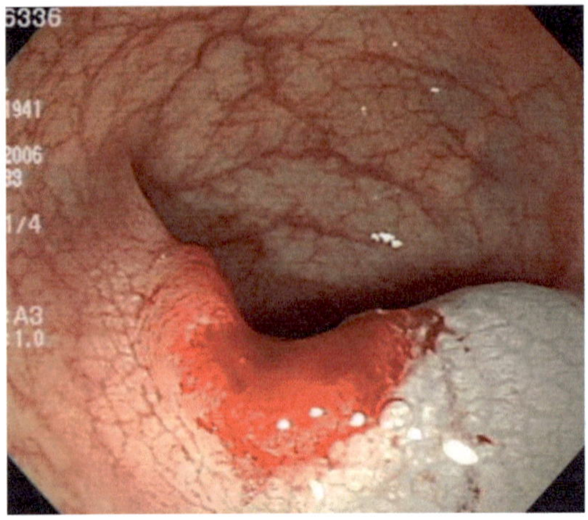

Fig. 4.3 Non-lifting sign; the lesion is not lifted by submucosal saline injection

4.5 Endoscopic Resection of Superficial Neoplastic Lesions

Endoscopic resection methods for superficial neoplastic lesions include snaring polypectomy, endoscopic mucosal resection (EMR), and endoscopic submucosal dissection (ESD). In choosing the endoscopic resection method, the size, endoscopic type, and predicted invasion depth of the lesion should be taken into consideration.

Snaring polypectomy should be only used for the pedunculated type. In snaring of pedunculated lesion, the snare should be placed near the base for acquiring enough resection margin.

Since endoscopic mucosal resection (EMR) was first described in 1973 as a strip biopsy technique, EMR is widely used for large polyp resection [20]. Clinically, EMR is the most commonly used method for endoscopic resection of superficial neoplastic lesions. However, in case of the larger sized lesion, it is difficult to acquiring en bloc resection by EMR. Practically, 2 cm may be the largest size that can be easily resected en bloc by EMR.

Endoscopic piecemeal mucosal resection (EPMR) could be used for larger sized lesions. If the superficial neoplastic lesions is suspected to be noninvasive, EPMR could be performed. But, it should be noted that EPMR is associated with a high incomplete resection rate and a high local recurrence rate [21].

As is well known, en bloc resection is desirable for accurate pathologic examinations, especially for evaluating the resection margin. Endoscopic submucosal dissection (ESD) is a new technique for en bloc resection of larger sized tumor. Since ESD was first contrived for gastric tumor resection, colorectal ESD was adopted later and is increasing now. Although colorectal ESD has not become a common method yet because of the difficult technique and high risk of complications, colorectal ESD can be safely performed by experienced experts [21, 22].

After endoscopic resection of superficial neoplastic lesions, the localization of the original lesion site may be necessary for colonoscopic surveillance or additional surgery. If a submucosal invasive cancer is suspected clinically, marking at the site of excision is recommended, using submucosal injection of India ink [23–25].

4.6 Pathologic Evaluation of Endoscopically Resected Superficial Neoplastic Lesions

The endoscopically resected specimens should be pinned to a board by pin immediately after resection, and soaked to 10% neutral buffered formalin to avoid shrinkage, autolysis or other tissue artifacts related to poor fixation (Fig. 4.4).

There has been controversy for the definition of a positive resection margin, and following three definitions are used commonly; (1) tumor cells present <1 mm from the transected margin, (2) tumor cells present <2 mm from the transected margin, and (3) tumor cells present within the diathermy of the transected margin [26–29].

Resection margin is more important in invasive lesions, and the status of vertical (deep) margin is more valuable than of lateral margin. If endoscopically resected T1 CRC shows a positie resection margin, additiona surgery should be considered.

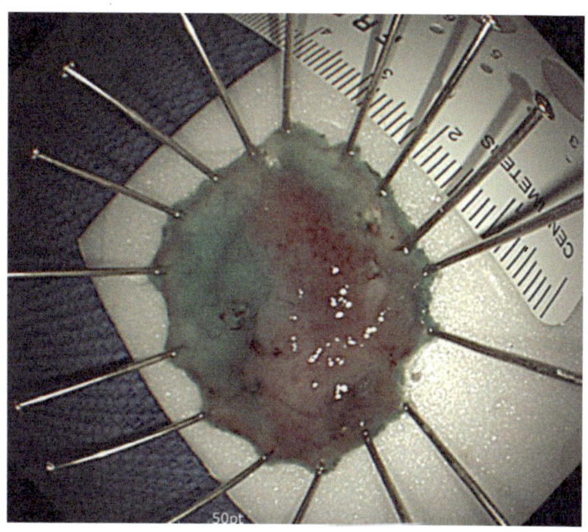

Fig. 4.4 Pinning of endoscopically resected specimen

Tis lesion has no risk of lymph node metastasis, so complete endoscopic resection of Tis is accepted as a curative therapy [30, 31].

However endoscopic resection of T1 CRC should be selectively applied because lymph node metastasis occurs in 7–15% [32–36]. Many previous researches reported the risk factors for LNM in T1 CRC, and commonly accepted pathologic risk factors for LNM in T1 CRC are deep submucosal invasion, vascular invasion, histopathologic high grade, and budding.

4.6.1 Deep Submucosal Invasion

Traditionally, for classification of the submucosal invasion depth (SM depth) levels, Haggit levels (level 1–4) for pedunculated lesion and Kikuchi levels (sm1–3) for sessile lesion were commonly used [33, 37, 38].

The Kikuchi level sm2/sm3 and the Haggit level 4 are regarded as the high risk for lymph node metastasis in T1 CRC.

On 2004, Kitajima, et al. proposed a new methods for measuring SM depth [39]. For sessile lesions, SM depth is measured from the lower border of the muscularis mucosae (MM) of the lesion, if the location of the MM is identified. If the location of the MM is not identified, the SM depth is measured from the surface of the lesion. For pedunculated lesions, SM depth is measured from the boundary line between the head and the stalk. When the deepest portion of invasion was limited in head (above Haggit level 2), the pedunculated lesions was defined as "a head invasion" and SM depth was regarded as 0 μm.

On 2012, Japanese Society for Cancer of the Colon and Rectum (JSCCR) proposed another method for measuring SM depth, in which method for pedunculated lesion is different [40]. For pedunculated lesions with a tangled MM, the SM depth invasion is measured from the boundary between the head and the stalk, same as in Kitajima's method. However, if the location of the MM is not identified in the pedunculated lesions, the SM depth is measured from the surface of the lesion. The concept of "head invasion" is same as that of Kitajima's method (Fig. 4.5).

The cut-off value between deep SM invasion and limited SM invasion is 1000 μm for sessile

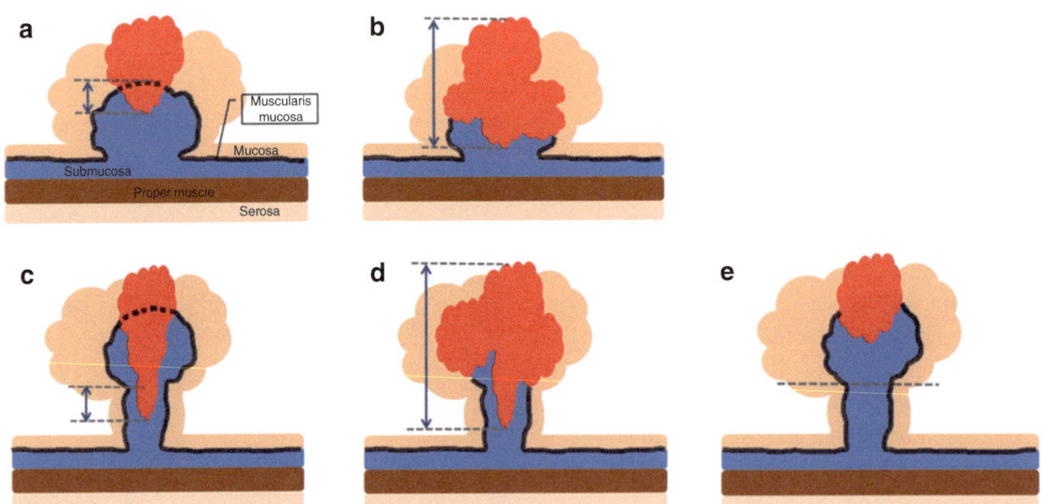

Fig. 4.5 Methods for measuring of SM depth. (**a**) Sessile lesion when MM identified. (**b**) Sessile lesion with MM not identified. (**c**) Pedunculated lesions with MM identified. (**d**) Pedunculated lesion with MM not identified. (**e**) Head invasion

lesions [12, 39, 40]. For pedunculated lesions, however, there is some dissent on the cut-off value between deep SM invasion and limited SM invasion. The level of the neck (Haggit level 2) has been usually accepted as the cut-off value between deep SM invasion and limited SM invasion. Kitaima, et al. proposed the 3000 μm of cut-off value between deep SM invasion and limited SM invasion [39]. According to JSCCR guidelines, the cut-off value between deep SM invasion and superficial SM invasion for pedunculated lesions is 1000 μm [40].

As stated above, identification of MM is very important for proper measuring the SM depth. However, it is often difficult to identify MM layer in specimen stained with hematoxylin and eosin. At this time, immunohistochemical stain of desmin might be helpful for identification of MM layer.

4.6.2 Vascular Invasion

Vascular invasion is a significant risk for lymph node and distant metastasis. An vascular invasion is defined as the presence of cancer cells within endothelial-lined channels. There are two types of vascular invasion, lymphatic invasion and venous invasion.

If cancer cells and cancer cell nests are present in the interstitial space and endothelial cells are identified around the space, lymphatic invasion can be concluded. Although endothelial cells are not identified, the presence of cancer cells in the interstitial may suggest lymphatic invasion (Fig. 4.6).

If cancer cell nests are presents surrounded by vascular wall structure such as vascular smooth muscle, venous invasion can be concluded (Fig. 4.7). If cancer cell nests are present in the vicinity of artery, venous invasion is strongly suggested.

However, it is often difficult to identify the vascular structure in specimens stained with hematoxylin and eosin. Special staining method such as elastic vas Gieson staining or Victoria staining are useful for evaluating venous invasion. Immunohistochemistry might be helpful for identifying lymphatic invasion (e.g. D2–40) and venous invasion (e.g. CD-34) [41, 42].

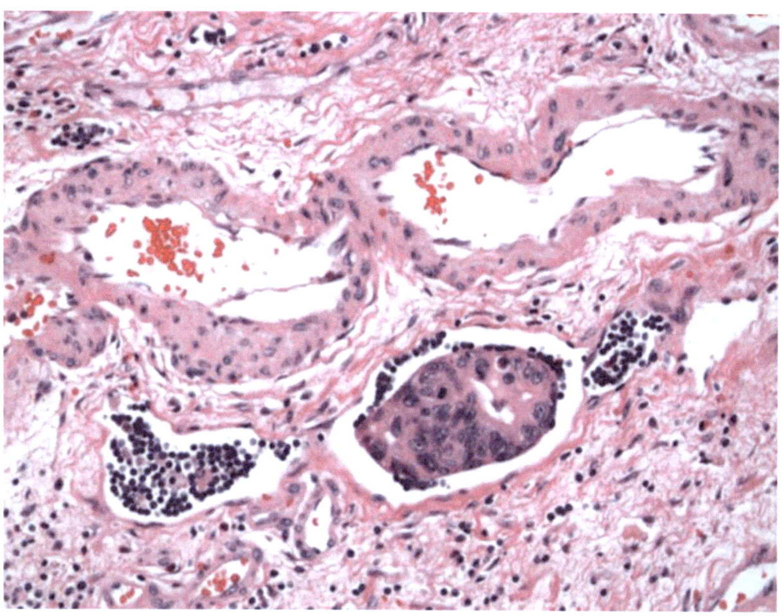

Fig. 4.6 Lymphatic invasion. Cancer cell nests are present in the interstitial space and endothelial cells are identified around the space

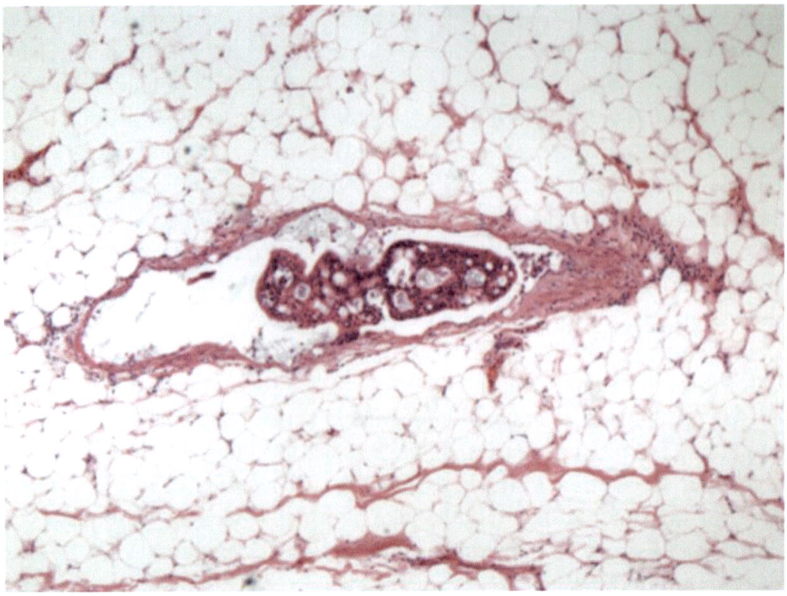

Fig. 4.7 Venous invasion. Cancer cell nests are presents surrounded by vascular smooth muscle

4.6.3 Histopathologic High Grade

Histopathologic high grade, such as poorly differentiated adenocarcinoma or signet ring cell carcinoma, is known as risk factor for lymph node metastasis.

According to modified criteria for WHO classification of adenocarcinoma, poorly differentiated adenocarcinoma is determined when the lesions show highly irregular glands, loss of glandular differentiation and loss of nuclear polarity [43]. Signet ring cell carcinoma and mucinous carcinoma are also regarded as unfavorable histologic type having the risk for lymph node metastasis in T1 CRC [28].

4.6.4 Tumor Budding

The budding (or sprouting) is defined as an cancer cell nest consisting of one or less than five cells that infiltrate the interstitium in the invasive front [28] (Fig. 4.8). If cancer cell nests show the feature of solid trabecular nests, consisting of five or more than five cells, it can be defined as "dedifferentiation". Depending on the number of budding viewed at ×200 magnification field, the grade of budding is classified into three grades; grade 1 (0–4), grade 2 (5–9), and grade 3 (10 or more). According to JSCCR guidelines, grade 1 is defined as "low grade" and grade 2/3 as "high grade". Several previous researches showed that high grade is an independent risk factor of lymph node metastasis in T1 CRC [36, 44]. However, budding is a relatively new concept, and is not yet world-widely accepted, because its reproducibility is criticized and the diagnostic criteria vary. And there is also a controversy that the its predicting value for lymph node metastasis is unproven, compared to other risk factors [45]. Further researches is need in this area.

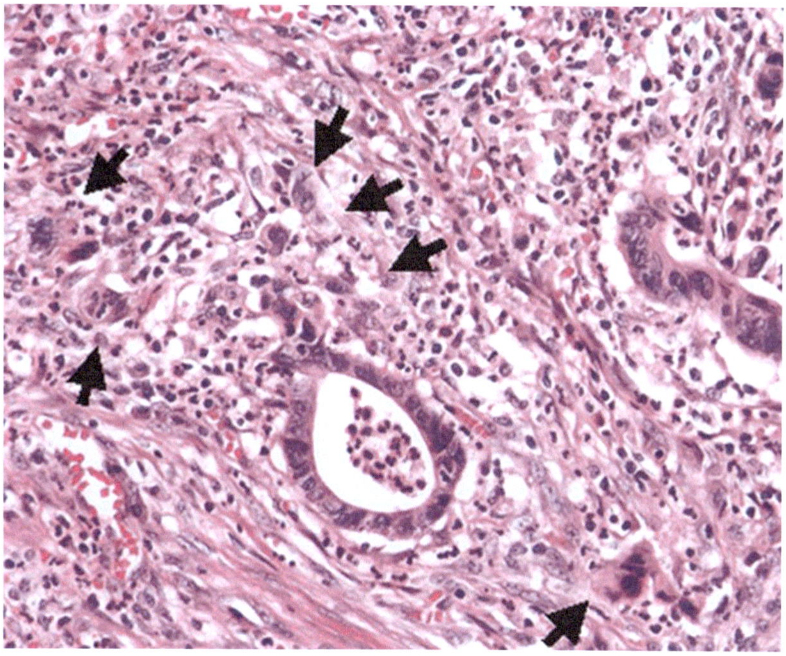

Fig. 4.8 Budding showing cancer cell nest consisting of one or less than five cells that infiltrate the interstitium in the invasive front

4.6.5 De Novo Cancer

The name of "de novo" cancer means that the cancer develop through new pathway which is different from adenoma-carcinoma sequence model [46–48]. The de novo cancers usually show relatively small size and surface depression. It has been estimated that about 22% of ECC developed by de novo carcinogenesis [49]. On the basis of pathologic features, de novo lesions show the absence of background adenoma, suggesting that the de novo cancer did not develop from an adenomatous precursor. Genetically, de novo colon cancers are known to lack of K-ras mutation [50, 51]. However, molecular genetics associated with de novo cancers remain largely unknown and the exact pathogenic mechanism associated with de novo cancer has not been determined, yet. Although the natural history of de novo cancer is largely unknown, these tumors may show more aggressive biologic behavior.

A previous research reported that the T1 CRC without background adenoma have several clinicopathologic characteristics of small size (<20 mm), flat or depressed type, deep SM depth and tumour budding, indicating that de novo cancers may have a more invasive potential [52]..

Although several researches reported that the absence of background adenoma might be the risk factor for lymph node metastasis in T1 CRC, there are not evidences enough to define the relationship between the absence of background adenoma and the risk of lymph node metastasis in T1 CRC [36, 52]. Further researches is need in this area.

4.7 Planning the Treatment Strategies for Superficial Neoplastic Lesions

If a superficial neoplastic lesion is found during colonoscopic examination, the first thing that should be done is to determine endoscopic respectability. Before determination of treatment planning, forcep biopsy should be avoided, because it may influence the nonlifting sign and cause false-positive event. Furthermore, pathologic diagnosis by biopsy (benign or malignancy) do not influence on treatment planning at all (surgery or endoscopic resection). So, that should be borne in mind "Never do biopsy before endoscopic resectability is totally determined". If biopsy was performed, endoscopic resection should be tried as soon as possible, because prolongation of the post-biopsy days can influence the nonlifting sign in endoscopically resectable lesions.

If the lesions is determined to be endoscopically resectable, endoscopic resection should be immediately tried without biopsy. Endoscopic resection is intended for both diagnosis and treatment. According to a previous research, it may be best that endoscopic resection be attempted within 3 weeks after biopsy [17].

If the lesions is determined to be endoscopically unresectable, biopsy should be done for histopathologic confirmation, and surgery may be considered.

After endoscopic resection, histopathologic evaluation of the resected specimen is performed, for determining the absence or the presence of risk factors. If the endoscopically resected lesions is confirmed to have risk factors (such as positive margin, deep submucosal invasion, vascular invasion, histopathologic high grade, and budding), additional surgery should be considered. If the endoscopically resected lesions is confirmed to have no risk factor, careful surveillance is enough without any more additional treatment (Fig. 4.9).

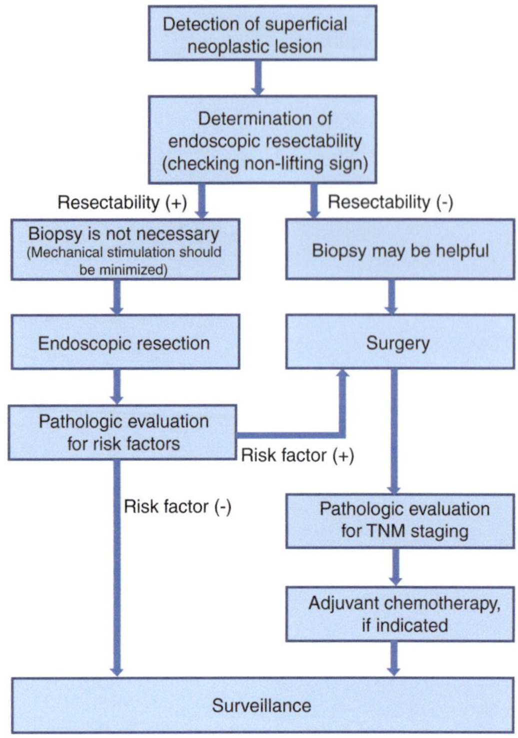

Fig. 4.9 Treatment strategies for superficial neoplastic lesions. The mechanical stimulation such as forceps biopsies should be minimized before endoscopic resection

4.8 Surveillance and Prognosis of Surgically or Endoscopically Resected Early Colorectal Cancer

4.8.1 Surveillance

For endoscopically resected Tis lesions with clear resection margin, colonoscopy surveillance is enough, not necessary for any other follow-up regimen, such as computed tomography or blood tests for carcinoembryonic antigen levels. In this case, colonoscopy surveillance in 1–3 years is recommended, and this follow-up regimen is based on polyp guidelines for high-risk adenoma [53–55].

If the resection margin of Tis lesion is not clear, colonoscopy surveillance should be performed 6 months to 1 year later for checking the development of local recurrence [40].

For endoscopically resected low-risk T1 lesions, the surveillance strategy for high-risk adenomas is regarded as to be appropriate follow-up. Based on the polyp guidelines, colonoscopy surveillance at 1 year is recommended. If advanced adenoma is detected in surveillance, repeated colonoscopy in 1 year is recommended. If no advanced adenoma is detected, repeated colonoscopy in 3 years then every 5 years is recommended [55, 56]. However, some recommend another more aggressive surveillance policy, similar to high-risk T1 lesions, including colonoscopy, computed tomography or blood tests for carcinoembryonic antigen levels [40].

For surgically resected high-risk T1 lesions, the same surveillance strategy as that of advanced CRC is recommended. It include colonoscopy (1, 3 years), blood tests for carcinoembryonic antigen levels (every 3 months in first 3 years, and then biannually in last 2 years), computed tomography (biannually in first 3 years, and then annually in last 2 years). For rectal cancer, the pelvis should be examined by computed tomography [40].

Although, additional completion surgery is strongly recommended for endoscopically resected high-risk T1 lesions, additional surgery might not be performed for special conditions. In this case, a more intensive surveillance strategy would be necessary for the increased risk of recurrence and timely salvage surgery. The polypectomy site should be closely followed, and biannual colonoscopic inspection for first 3 years is recommended. After this, surveillance policy for high-risk adenoma can be adopted. And other surveillance methods, such as computed tomography or tests for carcinoembryonic antigen levels, are also should be performed [55].

4.8.2 Prognosis

The survival of T1 CRC is known to be excellent. According to a project study by JSCCR, the recurrence rate of T1 CRC was approximately 1% [40]. However, the data about the long-term survival of endoscopically resected T1 CRC is still lack. According to several researches of Japan, the recurrence rate of endoscopically resected low-risk T1 CRC was 0.8–1% [57, 58]. However, the recurrence rate of endoscopically resected high-risk T1 CRC was significantly high to 6.6–13.5%, while the recurrence rate of surgically resected high-risk T1 CRC was less than 1%. This result strongly indicates the significance of additional surgery for endoscopically resected high-risk T1 CRC cases.

A recent research reported an interesting result [59]. Although the recurrence rate was significantly higher in endoscopically resected high-risk T1 CRC group than in surgically resected high-risk T1 CRC group, the overall survival was not significantly different between two groups (97% vs. 99%). This result may be caused by the recurrence patterns (local is more common recurrence pattern than distant) and successful salvage surgery, indicating the significance of intensive surveillance and early detection of recurrence.

References

1. Murakami T. Pathomorphological diagnosis. Definition and gross classification of early gastric cancer. Gann Monogr Cancer Res. 1971;11:53–5.
2. Muto T. Early colorectal cancer–concepts and clinical implications: introduction. World J Surg. 2000;24(9):1015.
3. Schlemper RJ, Riddell RH, Kato Y, Borchard F, Cooper HS, Dawsey SM, et al. The Vienna classification of gastrointestinal epithelial neoplasia. Gut. 2000; 47(2):251–5.
4. Dixon MF. Gastrointestinal epithelial neoplasia: Vienna revisited. Gut. 2002;51(1):130–1.
5. Weston AP, Campbell DR. Diminutive colonic polyps: histopathology, spatial distribution, concomitant significant lesions, and treatment complications. Am J Gastroenterol. 1995;90(1):24–8.
6. Lescher TC, Dockerty MB, Jackman RJ, Beahrs OH. Histopathology of the larger colonic polyp. Dis Colon Rectum. 1967;10(2):118–24.
7. Kudo S, Lambert R, Allen JI, Fujii H, Fujii T, Kashida H, et al. Nonpolypoid neoplastic lesions of the colorectal mucosa. Gastrointest Endosc. 2008;68 (4 Suppl):S3–47.
8. Wada Y, Kashida H, Kudo SE, Misawa M, Ikehara N, Hamatani S. Diagnostic accuracy of pit pattern and vascular pattern analyses in colorectal lesions. Dig Endosc. 2010;22(3):192–9.
9. Tanaka S, Sano Y. Aim to unify the narrow band imaging (NBI) magnifying classification for colorectal tumors: current status in Japan from a summary of the consensus symposium in the 79th Annual Meeting of the Japan Gastroenterological Endoscopy Society. Dig Endosc. 2011;23(Suppl 1):131–9.
10. Aiko T, Sasako M. The new Japanese Classification of Gastric Carcinoma: points to be revised. Gastric Cancer. 1998;1(1):25–30.
11. Japanese Gastric Cancer Association. Japanese classification of gastric carcinoma - 2nd English edition. Gastric Cancer. 1998;1(1):10–24.
12. The Paris endoscopic classification of superficial neoplastic lesions: esophagus, stomach, and colon: November 30 to December 1, 2002. Gastrointest Endosc. 2003;58(6 Suppl):S3–43.
13. Harada N, Hamada S, Kubo H, Oda S, Chijiiwa Y, Kabemura T, et al. Preoperative evaluation of submucosal invasive colorectal cancer using a 15-MHz ultrasound miniprobe. Endoscopy. 2001;33(3):237–40.

14. Hurlstone DP, Brown S, Cross SS, Shorthouse AJ, Sanders DS. Endoscopic ultrasound miniprobe staging of colorectal cancer: can management be modified? Endoscopy. 2005;37(8):710–4.
15. Fu KI, Sano Y, Kato S, Fujii T, Nagashima F, Yoshino T, et al. Chromoendoscopy using indigo carmine dye spraying with magnifying observation is the most reliable method for differential diagnosis between non-neoplastic and neoplastic colorectal lesions: a prospective study. Endoscopy. 2004;36(12):1089–93.
16. Uno Y, Munakata A. The non-lifting sign of invasive colon cancer. Gastrointest Endosc. 1994;40(4):485–9.
17. Han KS, Sohn DK, Choi DH, Hong CW, Chang HJ, Lim SB, et al. Prolongation of the period between biopsy and EMR can influence the nonlifting sign in endoscopically resectable colorectal cancers. Gastrointest Endosc. 2008;67(1):97–102.
18. Ishiguro A, Uno Y, Ishiguro Y, Munakata A, Morita T. Correlation of lifting versus non-lifting and microscopic depth of invasion in early colorectal cancer. Gastrointest Endosc. 1999;50(3):329–33.
19. Kato H, Haga S, Endo S, Hashimoto M, Katsube T, Oi I, et al. Lifting of lesions during endoscopic mucosal resection (EMR) of early colorectal cancer: implications for the assessment of resectability. Endoscopy. 2001;33(7):568–73.
20. Deyhle P, Largiader F, Jenny S. A method for endoscopic electroresection of sessile colonic polyps. Endoscopy. 1973;5:38–40.
21. Tanaka S, Oka S, Chayama K. Colorectal endoscopic submucosal dissection: present status and future perspective, including its differentiation from endoscopic mucosal resection. J Gastroenterol. 2008;43(9):641–51.
22. Lee EJ, Lee JB, Lee SH, Kim DS, Lee DH, Lee DS, et al. Endoscopic submucosal dissection for colorectal tumors–1,000 colorectal ESD cases: one specialized institute's experiences. Surg Endosc. 2013;27(1):31–9.
23. Elarini T, Wexner SD, Isenberg GA. The need for standardization of colonoscopic tattooing of colonic lesions. Dis Colon Rectum. 2015;58(2):264–7.
24. Hwang MR, Sohn DK, Park JW, Kim BC, Hong CW, Han KS, et al. Small-dose India ink tattooing for preoperative localization of colorectal tumor. J Laparoendosc Adv Surg Tech A. 2010;20(9):731–4.
25. Park JW, Sohn DK, Hong CW, Han KS, Choi DH, Chang HJ, et al. The usefulness of preoperative colonoscopic tattooing using a saline test injection method with prepackaged sterile India ink for localization in laparoscopic colorectal surgery. Surg Endosc. 2008;22(2):501–5.
26. Volk EE, Goldblum JR, Petras RE, Carey WD, Fazio VW. Management and outcome of patients with invasive carcinoma arising in colorectal polyps. Gastroenterology. 1995;109(6):1801–7.
27. Cooper HS, Deppisch LM, Gourley WK, Kahn EI, Lev R, Manley PN, et al. Endoscopically removed malignant colorectal polyps: clinicopathologic correlations. Gastroenterology. 1995;108(6):1657–65.
28. Ueno H, Mochizuki H, Hashiguchi Y, Shimazaki H, Aida S, Hase K, et al. Risk factors for an adverse outcome in early invasive colorectal carcinoma. Gastroenterology. 2004;127(2):385–94.
29. Seitz U, Bohnacker S, Seewald S, Thonke F, Brand B, Braiutigam T, et al. Is endoscopic polypectomy an adequate therapy for malignant colorectal adenomas? Presentation of 114 patients and review of the literature. Dis Colon Rectum. 2004;47(11):1789–96, discussion 96–7.
30. Morson BC, Whiteway JE, Jones EA, Macrae FA, Williams CB. Histopathology and prognosis of malignant colorectal polyps treated by endoscopic polypectomy. Gut. 1984;25(5):437–44.
31. Kyzer S, Begin LR, Gordon PH, Mitmaker B. The care of patients with colorectal polyps that contain invasive adenocarcinoma. Endoscopic polypectomy or colectomy? Cancer. 1992;70(8):2044–50.
32. Tominaga K, Nakanishi Y, Nimura S, Yoshimura K, Sakai Y, Shimoda T. Predictive histopathologic factors for lymph node metastasis in patients with nonpedunculated submucosal invasive colorectal carcinoma. Dis Colon Rectum. 2005;48(1):92–100.
33. Kikuchi R, Takano M, Takagi K, Fujimoto N, Nozaki R, Fujiyoshi T, et al. Management of early invasive colorectal cancer. Risk of recurrence and clinical guidelines. Dis Colon Rectum. 1995;38(12):1286–95.
34. Sohn DK, Chang HJ, Park JW, Choi DH, Han KS, Hong CW, et al. Histopathological risk factors for lymph node metastasis in submucosal invasive colorectal carcinoma of pedunculated or semipedunculated type. J Clin Pathol. 2007;60(8):912–5.
35. Okabe S, Shia J, Nash G, Wong WD, Guillem JG, Weiser MR, et al. Lymph node metastasis in T1 adenocarcinoma of the colon and rectum. J Gastrointest Surg. 2004;8(8):1032–9, discussion 1039–40.
36. Suh JH, Han KS, Kim BC, Hong CW, Sohn DK, Chang HJ, et al. Predictors for lymph node metastasis in T1 colorectal cancer. Endoscopy. 2012;44(6):590–5.
37. Haggitt RC, Glotzbach RE, Soffer EE, Wruble LD. Prognostic factors in colorectal carcinomas arising in adenomas: implications for lesions removed by endoscopic polypectomy. Gastroenterology. 1985;89(2):328–36.
38. Kudo S. Endoscopic mucosal resection of flat and depressed types of early colorectal cancer. Endoscopy. 1993;25(7):455–61.
39. Kitajima K, Fujimori T, Fujii S, Takeda J, Ohkura Y, Kawamata H, et al. Correlations between lymph node metastasis and depth of submucosal invasion in submucosal invasive colorectal carcinoma: a Japanese collaborative study. J Gastroenterol. 2004;39(6):534–43.
40. Watanabe T, Itabashi M, Shimada Y, Tanaka S, Ito Y, Ajioka Y, et al. Japanese Society for Cancer of the Colon and Rectum (JSCCR) guidelines 2010 for the treatment of colorectal cancer. Int J Clin Oncol. 2012;17(1):1–29.

41. Shieh YS, Lee HS, Shiah SG, Chu YW, Wu CW, Chang LC. Role of angiogenic and non-angiogenic mechanisms in oral squamous cell carcinoma: correlation with histologic differentiation and tumor progression. J Oral Pathol Med. 2004;33(10):601–6.
42. Agarwal D, Pardhe N, Bajpai M, Gupta S, Mathur N, Vanaki SS, et al. Characterization, localization and patterning of lymphatics and blood vessels in oral squamous cell carcinoma: a comparative study using D2-40 and CD-34 IHC marker. J Clin Diagn Res. 2014;8(10):ZC86–9.
43. WHO. Histological typing of intestinal tumours. In: Jass JR, Sobin LH, editors. World Health Organisation international histological classification of tumours. Berlin: Springer; 1989.
44. Masaki T, Matsuoka H, Sugiyama M, Abe N, Sakamoto A, Atomi Y. Actual number of tumor budding as a new tool for the individualization of treatment of T1 colorectal carcinomas. J Gastroenterol Hepatol. 2006;21(7):1115–21.
45. Prall F. Tumour budding in colorectal carcinoma. Histopathology. 2007;50(1):151–62.
46. Vogelstein B, Fearon ER, Hamilton SR, Kern SE, Preisinger AC, Leppert M, et al. Genetic alterations during colorectal-tumor development. N Engl J Med. 1988;319(9):525–32.
47. Kuramoto S, Oohara T. Minute cancers arising de novo in the human large intestine. Cancer. 1988;61(4):829–34.
48. Shimoda T, Ikegami M, Fujisaki J, Matsui T, Aizawa S, Ishikawa E. Early colorectal carcinoma with special reference to its development de novo. Cancer. 1989;64(5):1138–46.
49. Goto H, Oda Y, Murakami Y, Tanaka T, Hasuda K, Goto S, et al. Proportion of de novo cancers among colorectal cancers in Japan. Gastroenterology. 2006; 131(1):40–6.
50. Umetani N, Sasaki S, Masaki T, Watanabe T, Matsuda K, Muto T. Involvement of APC and K-ras mutation in non-polypoid colorectal tumorigenesis. Br J Cancer. 2000;82(1):9–15.
51. Yashiro M, Carethers JM, Laghi L, Saito K, Slezak P, Jaramillo E, et al. Genetic pathways in the evolution of morphologically distinct colorectal neoplasms. Cancer Res. 2001;61(6):2676–83.
52. Han KS, Lim SW, Sohn DK, Chang HJ, Oh JH, Lee JH, et al. Clinicopathological characteristics of T1 colorectal cancer without background adenoma. Color Dis. 2013;15(3):e124–9.
53. Davila RE, Rajan E, Baron TH, Adler DG, Egan JV, Faigel DO, et al. ASGE guideline: colorectal cancer screening and surveillance. Gastrointest Endosc. 2006;63(4):546–57.
54. Lieberman DA, Rex DK, Winawer SJ, Giardiello FM, Johnson DA, Levin TR, et al. Guidelines for colonoscopy surveillance after screening and polypectomy: a consensus update by the US Multi-Society Task Force on Colorectal Cancer. Gastroenterology. 2012;143(3):844–57.
55. Steele RJ, Pox C, Kuipers EJ, Minoli G, Lambert R, International Agency for Research on Cancer. European guidelines for quality assurance in colorectal cancer screening and diagnosis. First edition–management of lesions detected in colorectal cancer screening. Endoscopy. 2012;44(Suppl 3):SE140–50.
56. Benson AB III, Venook AP, Bekaii-Saab T, Chan E, Chen YJ, Cooper HS, et al. Colon cancer, version 3.2014. J Natl Compr Canc Netw. 2014;12(7):1028–59.
57. Ikematsu H, Yoda Y, Matsuda T, Yamaguchi Y, Hotta K, Kobayashi N, et al. Long-term outcomes after resection for submucosal invasive colorectal cancers. Gastroenterology. 2013;144(3):551–9, quiz e14.
58. Yoshii S, Nojima M, Nosho K, Omori S, Kusumi T, Okuda H, et al. Factors associated with risk for colorectal cancer recurrence after endoscopic resection of T1 tumors. Clin Gastroenterol Hepatol. 2014;12(2):292–302.e3.
59. Nam MJ, Han KS, Kim BC, Hong CW, Sohn DK, Chang HJ, et al. Long-term outcomes of locally or radically resected T1 colorectal cancer. Color Dis. 2016;18(9):852–60.

5 Management of Colorectal Bleeding

Chang Won Hong

Common causes of colorectal bleeding are diverticulosis, hemorrhoids, and ischemic colitis. Less common causes include post-polypectomy ulcers, colorectal neoplasms, inflammatory bowel diseases, colon angiodysplasia and rectal ulcer [1, 2]. Most often colorectal bleeding (hematochezia) is self-limited and does not require urgent intervention or hospitalization. But if there are re-bleeding events or large amount bleeding, we need to have diagnostic and therapeutic approach, resuscitation, exclusion of upper gastrointestinal bleeding, colon preparation, and colonoscopic intervention.

To perform a successful colonoscopic intervention in case of hematochezia, adequate colon preparation and appropriate selection of hemostatic method are needed. Colon cleansing is an essential step before the emergency colonoscopy, although it takes time. This chapter provides an overview of the techniques and accessories used during colonoscopic procedures for colorectal bleeding.

Postpolypectomy bleeding is the most common complication of colonoscopic polypectomy [3]. Bleeding occurs after polypectomy because a submucosal artery is either not sealed or the seal is opened later. Postpolypectomy bleeding is described as immediate or delayed. Large and broad based colonic polyps have a greater risk of immediate and delayed postpolypectomy bleeding. Pedunculated polyps with a thick stalk have also high risk [4].

Several endoscopic techniques have been proposed to prevent or to control postpolypectomy bleeding, such as APC (Argon Plasma Coagulation), clipping, ligation, injection (Figs. 5.1 and 5.2).

5.1 APC (Argon Plasma Coagulation)

5.1.1 The Principle of APC

When a probe emitting gas is placed at an adequate distance from a tissue and high-frequency voltage is applied between the probe and the tissue, the gas between the probe and the tissue becomes ionized and electrically conductive. If the gas between the probe and the tissue is a noble gas (argon, helium, etc.), an electric strength for ionization is 500 V/mm. Among the noble gases, argon is relatively cheap, argon is preferred. The ionized argon gas forms argon plasma beams. It can be visualized as sparks. Argon plasma beams conduct the high-frequency current to the tissue, and result in coagulation and drying. The thermal effect of APC is limited to the devitalized

C.W. Hong, M.D., Ph.D.
National Cancer Center, Goyang-si, Gyeonggi-do, South Korea
e-mail: hong@ncc.re.kr

D.K. Sohn (ed.), *Practice and Principles in Therapeutic Colonoscopy*,
https://doi.org/10.1007/978-3-662-46552-3_5

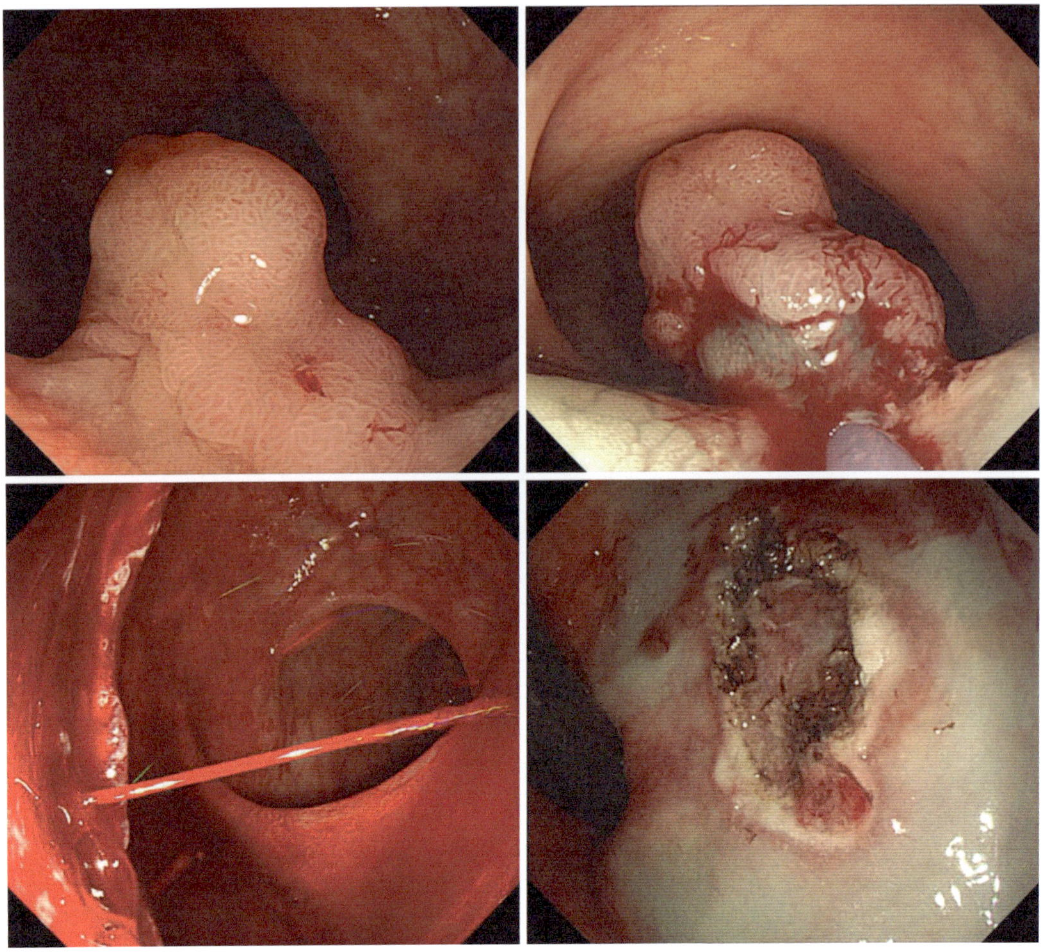

Fig. 5.1 Immediate bleeding after polypectomy can be easily controlled by coagulation

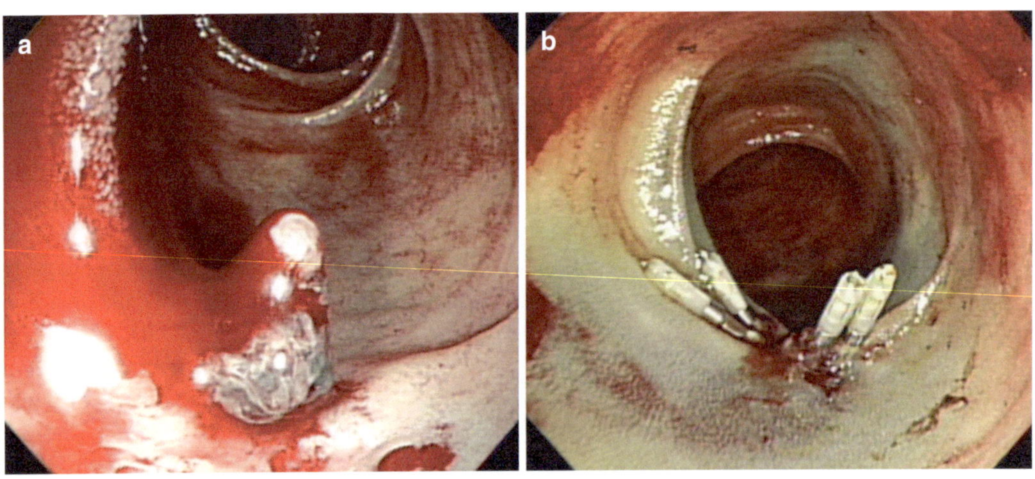

Fig. 5.2 (**a**) Active bleeding site covered with blood clots, (**b**) bleeding control by clipping

tissue. The electrically active argon beams are directed from the probe to electrically conductive tissue closest to the probe. After the target tissue becomes dry and loses conductivity, the argon beams move from dry tissue to wet tissue. Because of the loss of conductivity at a treated tissue, the depth of drying, coagulation, devitalization is limited [5–7].

5.1.2 Equipment of APC

Argon plasma coagulator is consisted of argon tank, flow valves, probe and electrosurgical generator (Fig. 5.3). The argon tank is a cylinder with a pressure-reducing valve. Argon tank must have automatically controlled flow rates and limitation of the pressure.

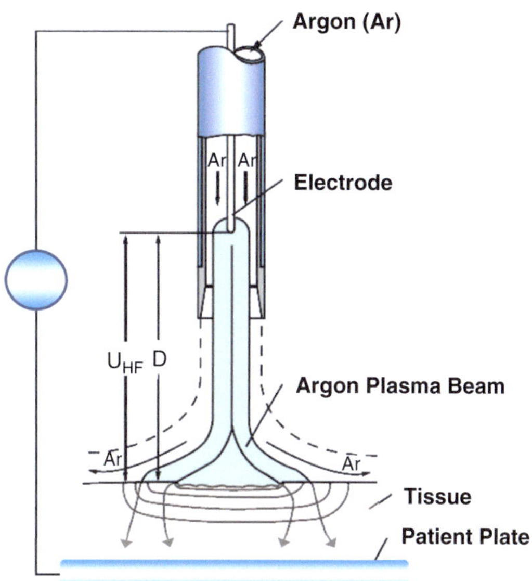

Fig. 5.3 Principles of Argon Plasma Coagulator (APC)

An APC probe for endoscopy consists of a nonconductive flexible tube. The distal end of APC probe has electrode which is connected to the high-frequency generator by a wire within the lumen of flexible tube (Fig. 5.4). For safety, the electrode is receded from the distal end of the tube so that it cannot contact with tissue (Fig. 5.5).

An electrosurgical generator must be a high-frequency current source so that it must provide sufficiently high voltage for the ionization of argon.

The depth of coagulation depends on setting, application time and application technique. For a shallower depth, movement of activated probe tip is needed. If the activated probe is not moved for about 3–10 s, the depth of thermal effect is up to about 2 mm. Over 10 s, the depth of thermal effect increases to about 3–4 mm.

5.2 Endoscopic Clips

Endoscopic clip and clipping devices are designed to accomplish approximation of tissues during endoscopy [8–11]. Metallic clipping devices were first introduced for the primary purpose of achieving hemostasis of focal gastrointestinal bleeding. A successful deployment of the clip for hemostasis of postpolypectomy bleeding is very effective [12]. It results in immediate and complete cessation of bleeding. But a precise targeting is required for

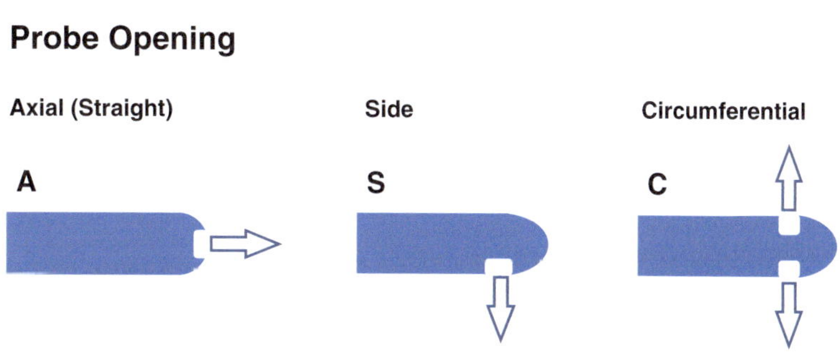

Fig. 5.4 Various types of APC probe

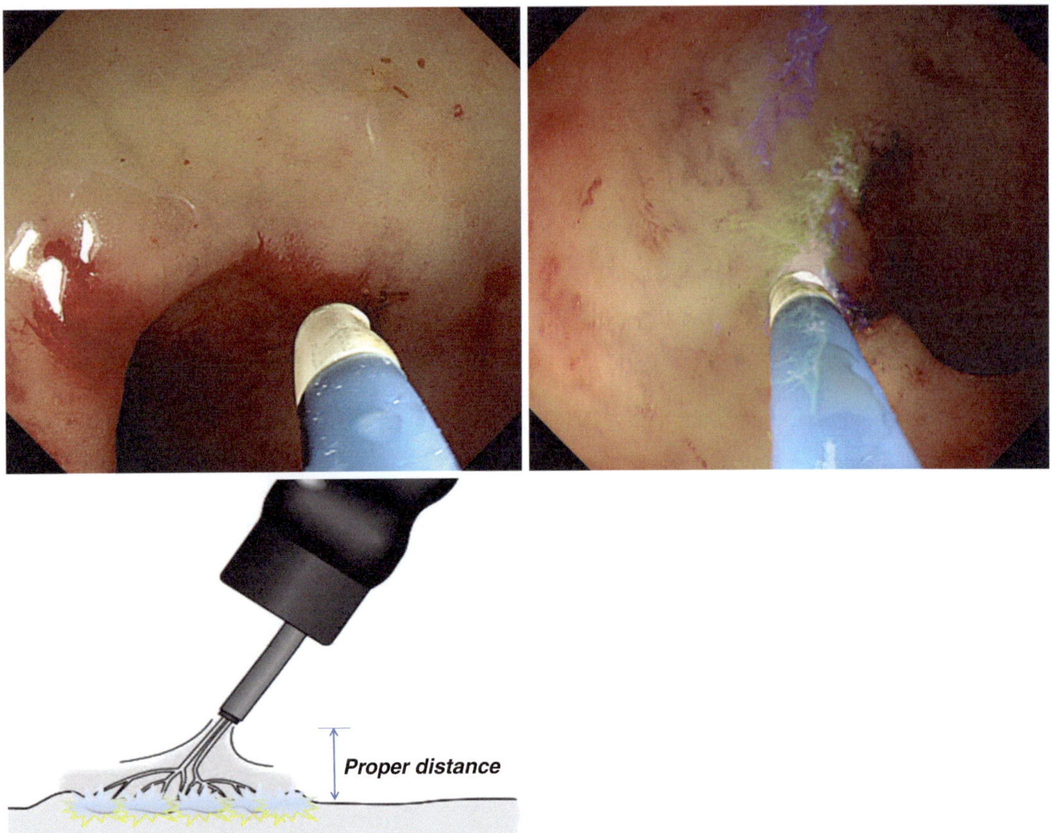

Fig. 5.5 The distal end of APC probe should not be contacted with tissues

a successful clipping. In a major bleeding when large amount of blood obscure the view, epinephrine injection will usually slow bleeding to allow accurate targeting. Irrigation with water pump and suctioning of clot are important too.

5.2.1 Equipment

Several endoscopic clipping devices are commercially available. All devices have two components: metallic clips and deployment catheter-handle. Clips are double or triple pronged metals. The clip fixing device consists of a control section and insertion tube. The control section is a plastic parts that manipulate clip loading and firing. With the rotatable version, a rotator disk located on the control section and is used to turn the clip to the desired orientation. The insertion tube is made up of a metal coil and outer plastic sheath. At a distal end of the metal coil, there is a hooking apparatus for attaching of clip. The length of insertion tube is up to 230 cm.

The clips are basically multiangled stainless-steel ribbon. Standard hemoclips is measured 6 mm in length and 1.2 mm in width. The clips are available in several lengths (short/standard/long) and have an opening angle of 90° or 135°. Clips open from 6 to 12 mm, depending on the specific type.

Several endoscopic clips are currently available. (EZ clip and QuickClip (Olympus Medical, Tokyo, Japan), Resolution Clip (Microvasive Endoscopy, Boston Scientific Inc., Natick, MA, USA), Triclip (Cook Endoscopy, Winston-Salem, NC, USA), Multi-Clip (InScope Inc., a Division of Ethicon Endosurgery, Cincinnati, Ohio) (Fig. 5.6).

A single use clip-deploying device (QuickClip) with a preloaded clip offsets the need for clip loading. Its configuration and function are otherwise similar to the reusable device, though it lacks the clip rotator in its original model. The QuickClip opens to 6 mm. A further modification on the single-use clipping device (QuickClip 2) includes the rotating mechanism, with a prong opening of 9.5 mm. A newly developed QuickClip Pro has open-and-close function to facilitate correct positioning prior to deployment. The arms can be closed, reopened and repositioned. QuickClip Pro includes the rotating mechanism, and can open to 11 mm. The QuickClip Pro is suitable for use in magnetic resonance (MR) environments.

A second single-use, preloaded clipping device (Resolution Clip) deploys a 2-pronged

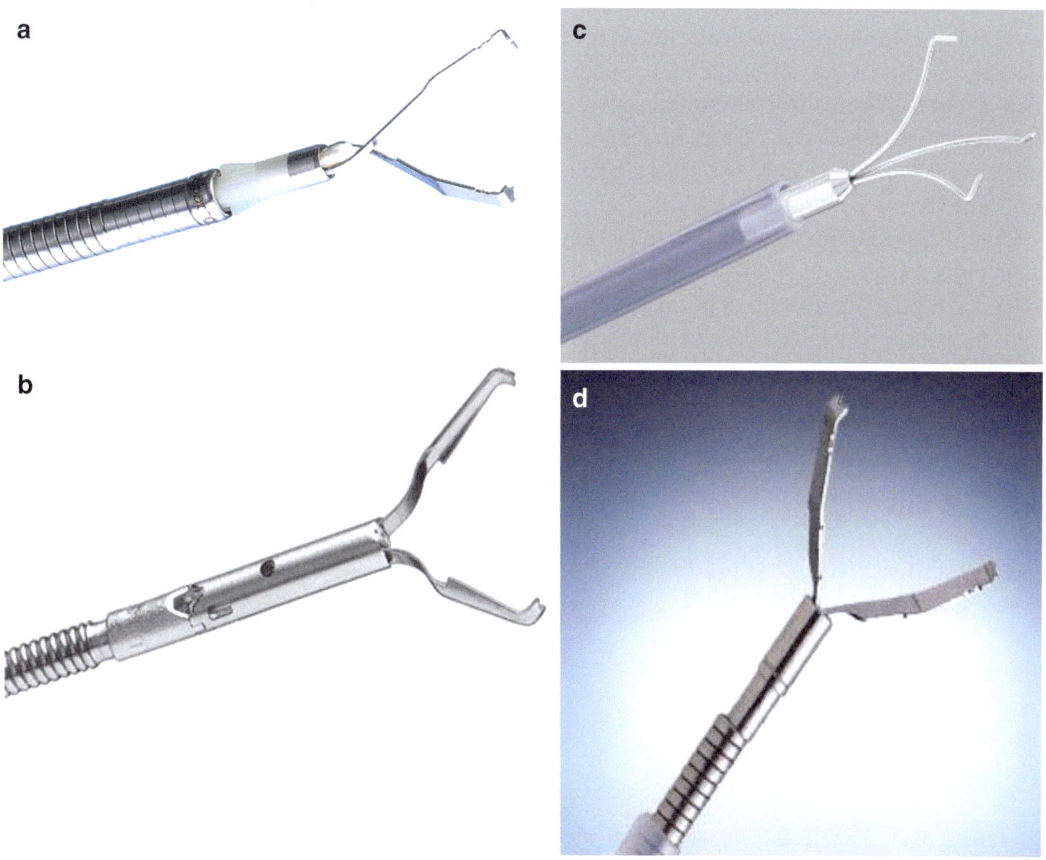

Fig. 5.6 Endoscopic clip. (**a**) EZ clip, (**b**) Resolution clip, (**c**) Triclip, (**d**) Quickclip2

stainless steel clip that tapers from 1.9 to 1.2 mm in width from base to tip and opens to a maximum of 11 mm. It is offered in 155 and 235 cm lengths and can be used through a 2.8 mm endoscope accessory channel. A unique characteristic of the Resolution Clip is the ability to reopen and reposition the clip after closing, up to five times as long as the device has not been fully fired.

Another single-use clipping device (TriClip) delivers a 3-pronged stainless steel clip preloaded on either a 7 or 8F catheter with a disposable handle. The 8F devices have an port for flushing the field. The clip opens to a maximum diameter of 12 mm. The clip is withdrawn into the sheath to allow passage through the endoscope accessory channel. The firing mechanism re-exposes the clip from the sheath, opens it to its maximum diameter, closes it onto the target tissue, and disconnects the clip.

EZ clip is primarily marketed in Japan and part of Asia. It has the advantage of a reloadable deployment device so that several clips of varying arm length of between 5.0 and 8.5 mm. Distal angles of 90° or 135° can be used in a single setting with the same fixing device.

Multi-Clip is nearing distribution. It can apply four clips sequentially without reloading. This device grasp the tissue with apposing arms of a forceps before clip application. The clips can also be rotated, closed, reopened, and repositioned for optimal application.

5.2.2 Indications

Hemostasis for

(a) Mucosal/submucosal defects
(b) Bleeding ulcers
(c) Bleeding arteries <2 mm in size
(d) Polypectomy sites
(e) Diverticula in the colon

Endoscopic clipping is safe and effective for hemostatic therapy of postpolypectomy bleeding and other bleeding lesions. Initial failure of clip placement may be due to inability to achieve proper orientation or inability to grasp fibrotic hard tissue. Orientation challenges are diminished by using the rotatable devices. If there is a vessel within an ulcer with a large fibrotic base, there may not be adequate tissue to anchor a clip device. Malfunction of the reusable clip-fixing device is frequently due to improper clip loading. Through ex vivo training, familiarity with device loading, delivery, and deployment may be obtained. And safe and successful application will be possible [12].

5.3 Endoloop (Ligation)

The risk of bleeding is greater with large broad based polyps or large polyps with thick stalks. Several endoscopic techniques have been developed to prevent bleeding. Injection of the stalk with epinephrine solution or sclerosing agents before cutting is recommended to diminish the risk of postpolypectomy bleeding. However, epinephrine injection may prevent only procedural bleeding, and sclerosing agents injection may increase the risk of perforation. The use of an endoloop may minimize the risk for bleeding after endoscopic polypectomy of large pedunculated colorectal polyps [8–10, 13, 14].

5.3.1 Equipment

A detachable snare (endoloop) system is composed of an operating part and an attached loop (Fig. 5.7). The operating part consists of a Teflon sheath 2.5 mm in diameter and 195 cm in working length, a stainless steel coil sheath 1.9 mm in diameter, a hook wire (to which the loop is attached), and a handle. Endoloops are currently available in diameters of 20 and 30 mm (MAJ-340 and MAJ-254; Olympus Medical, Tokyo, Japan). The larger loop can be opened to a size of 50 by 30 mm. Endoloops are composed with a nonconductive sliding nylon loop and reusable plastic sheath with operating handle. Elliptical- or circular-shaped soft Teflon ring is heattreated and a silicon rubber stopper maintains the tightness of the loop. Some older devices required preloading of the loop onto the hook wire. The loop is advanced out of the sheath and placed around the target tissue, usually the stalk of a large

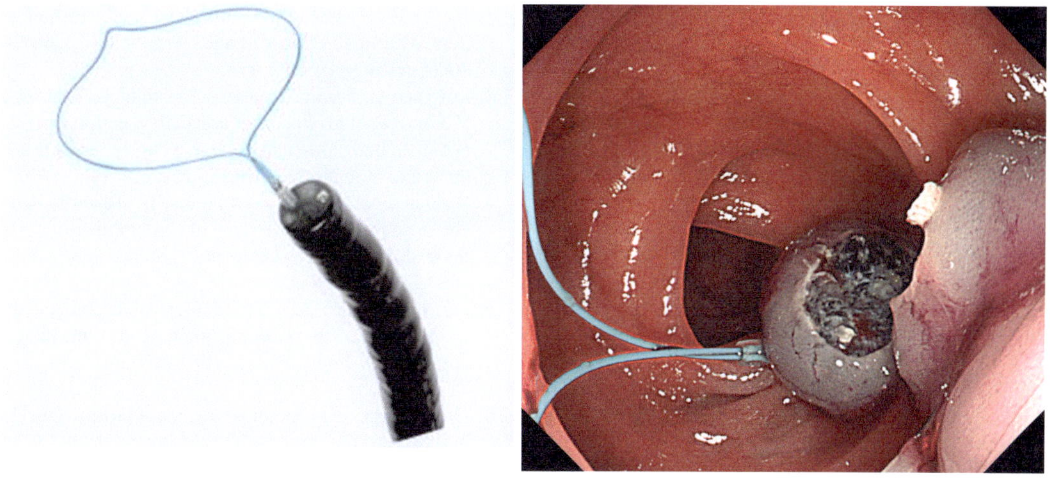

Fig. 5.7 (**a**) Endoloop, (**b**) An endoloop was firstly applied to resect a large-stalk polyp without bleeding

pedunculated polyp. The loop is tightened with advancement of a silicon rubber stopper by using the handle. When the loop is closed to the desired extent, as an evidence tissue cyanosis or hemostasis is seen, it is then released from the hook wire. There is a loop-cutting device that can be used to cut and release the nylon loop if it is malpositioned or fails to release from the catheter.

5.3.2 Clinical Use

Before application, the loop is retracted inside the plastic sheath for insertion through the accessory channel of the colonoscope. Using a large-channel therapeutic endoscope is preferred because that provides adequate suction alongside the sheath. After the loop had been extended and applied at the base of the stalk, it was tightened around the stalk by sliding the stopper with handle, then detached from the operating part. To ensure sufficient tightening, observe the color of the polyp head changing to dark red (cyanotic) after ligation. A diathermic snare then is used to cut the stalk of the polyp above the tightened loop. The satisfactory position of the endoloop is low on the stalk, to allow room to place the electrocautery snare between the endoloop and the polyp head.

Detachable loop ligating devices have been associated with loop entanglement with snare complicating polypectomy, slippage of the loop resulting in delayed bleeding, and inadvertent transection of the polyp stalk leading to immediate bleeding. Optimal positioning of a loop device, adequate tightening and optimal cutting of stalk generally requires more experience relative to standard diagnostic endoscopic techniques.

5.4 Injection

Injection of an epinephrine solution into the polyp stalk reduces the blood flow and promotes vasoconstriction and compression. Epinephrine injection is the most commonly used method of preventing bleeding in pedunculated polyps because it is less difficult and less expensive to use [8, 10, 15].

5.4.1 Equipment

Injection needles consist of an outer sheath (plastic, Teflon, or stainless steel) and an inner hollow-core needle (19–25 gauge) (Fig. 5.8). The needle tip is typically beveled. Length of needle tip should be sufficient to penetrate through the submucosa and not so long as to penetrate colon serosa. The diameter of outer sheath is from 2.3 to 2.8 mm. Most commercially available injection needles are single-use, disposable devices. Metal coil sheathed needles

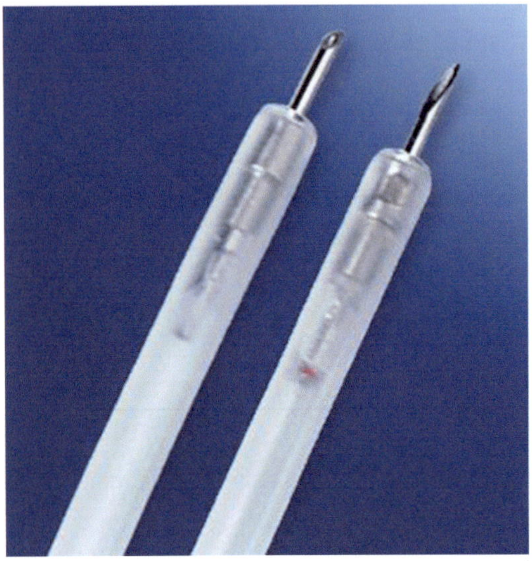

Fig. 5.8 Injection needle

may offer advantages over plastic sheathed needles in that they are less to kink and more apt to fully functional when in coiled colonoscope (in excessive looping condition or J-turn position).

5.4.2 Clinical Use

Using a handle on the end of the needle sheath, the operator can retract the needle into the sheath for safe passage through the working channel of the endoscope. When the catheter is placed near the target tissue, the needle can be extended out of the end of the sheath to a preset distance, and a syringe attached to the handle is used to inject liquid agents into the target tissue. Injection of various solutions including epinephrine (1:10,000 - 1:100,000) achieves hemostasis by both mechanical tamponade and cytochemical mechanisms.

References

1. Kovacs T, Jensen D. Acute lower gastrointestinal bleeding. In: Weinstein W, Hawkey C, Bosch J, editors. Clinical gastroenterology and hepatology. London: Elsevier Mosby; 2005. p. 127–31.
2. Jensen D, Machicado G. Where to look and how to treat diverticular hemorrhage. Am J Gastroenterol. 2006;101(Suppl):S202, 474.
3. Luigiano C, Ferrara F, Ghersi S, Fabbri C, Cennamo V, Landi P, et al. Endoclip-assisted resection of large pedunculated colorectal polyps: technical aspects and outcome. Dig Dis Sci. 2010;55(6):1726–31.
4. Macrae FA, Tan KG, Williams CB. Towards safer colonoscopy: a report on the complications of 5000 diagnostic or therapeutic colonoscopies. Gut. 1983;24(5):376–83.
5. Farin G, Grund KE. Technology of argon plasma coagulation with particular regard to endoscopic applications. Endosc Surg Allied Technol. 1994;2(1): 71–7.
6. Grund KE. Argon plasma coagulation (APC): ballyhoo or breakthrough? Endoscopy. 1997;29(3): 196–8.
7. Farin G, Grund K. Priciples of electrosurgery, laser, and argon plasma coagulation with particular regard to colonoscopy. In: Colonoscopy; principles and practice. 2nd ed. Hoboken: Wiley-Blackwell; 2009. p. 328–45.
8. Ginsberg G. Accessories. In: Colonoscopy; principles and practice. 2nd ed. Hoboken: Wiley-Blackwell; 2009. p. 306–17.
9. Michael J, Stephen J. Clips, loops, and bands: applications in the colon. In: Colonoscopy; principles and practice. 2nd ed. Hoboken: Wiley-Blackwell; 2009. p. 306–17.
10. Asge Technology Committee, Conway JD, Adler DG, Diehl DL, Farraye FA, Kantsevoy SV, et al. Endoscopic hemostatic devices. Gastrointest Endosc. 2009;69(6):987–96.
11. Technology Assessment Committee, Chuttani R, Barkun A, Carpenter S, Chotiprasidhi P, Ginsberg GG, et al. Endoscopic clip application devices. Gastrointest Endosc. 2006;63(6):746–50.
12. Cipolletta L, Bianco MA, Rotondano G, Catalano M, Prisco A, De Simone T. Endoclip-assisted resection of large pedunculated colon polyps. Gastrointest Endosc. 1999;50(3):405–6.
13. Iishi H, Tatsuta M, Narahara H, Iseki K, Sakai N. Endoscopic resection of large pedunculated colorectal polyps using a detachable snare. Gastrointest Endosc. 1996;44(5):594–7.
14. Katsinelos P, Kountouras J, Paroutoglou G, Beltsis A, Chatzimavroudis G, Zavos C, et al. Endoloop-assisted polypectomy for large pedunculated colorectal polyps. Surg Endosc. 2006;20(8):1257–61.
15. Lee SH, Chung IK, Kim SJ, Kim JO, Ko BM, Kim WH, et al. Comparison of postpolypectomy bleeding between epinephrine and saline submucosal injection for large colon polyps by conventional polypectomy: a prospective randomized, multicenter study. World J Gastroenterol. 2007;13(21):2973–7.

Management of Colonic Obstruction

6

Byung Chang Kim

6.1 Stent Placements for Malignant Obstruction

6.1.1 Introduction

The causes of pathological colonic obstruction are colorectal neoplasms and complications of diverticular diseases and inflammatory bowel diseases. This chapter mainly introduced the management of colorectal obstruction with malignant and short describe ballooning for benign stricture.

About 7–30% of the patients with primary colorectal cancer (CRC) present with obstructive symptoms like abdominal distension, nausea and vomiting [1, 2]. In CRC with obstruction, emergency surgical colorectal resection is usually avoided because surgical decompression (including stomy and bypass surgery) is associated with high morbidity (45–50%) and mortality (15–20%) [3–6]. In addition, permanent stoma creation has a negative impact on patients' quality of life and increase the cost of stomy care [7].

Since the first palliative use of metal stents in the early 1990s [8, 9], there has been rapidly increased the application of self-expanding metal stents (SEMS) for palliative care for malignant colorectal obstruction [10–14]. SEMS insertion for malignant colorectal obstruction can decompress the colorectal obstruction, clean the bowel, precise investigate the distant or loco-regional metastasis, and evaluate the entire colon for synchronous neoplasm. SEMS are popularly used as a non-surgical alternative for the "palliation" of intestinal obstruction and a "bridge to surgery" to permit one stage surgery in the latest date. The clinical outcomes of SEMS insertion are composed by technical success and clinical success in malignant obstruction. Technical success is defined as the appropriate placement of stent across the stenosis site. Clinical success is defined as the regression of symptoms and signs of obstruction within 48 h after SEMS insertion [15]. Two systematic reviews reported the technical success rate of 66.6–100% and the clinical success rate of 46–100% [16, 17].

SEMS insertion for colorectal obstruction as a bridge to elective surgery is not recommended as a standard treatment of symptomatic left-sided malignant colorectal obstruction [18, 19]. However, SEMS placements as a bridge to surgery may be considered as an alternative treatment option in patients with potentially curable obstructive colorectal cancer as high surgical risk (i.e. ASA $\geq$ III and/or age > 70 years) because they have an increased risk of post-operative mortality [18, 19]. An

B.C. Kim, M.D.
National Cancer Center, Goyang-si, Gyeonggi-do, South Korea
e-mail: mdzara@ncc.re.kr

D.K. Sohn (ed.), *Practice and Principles in Therapeutic Colonoscopy*,
https://doi.org/10.1007/978-3-662-46552-3_6

optimal interval to operation of 5–10 days is recommended when SEMS is used as a bridge to elective surgery in patients with potentially curable left-sided colon cancer [18]. SEMS placement is the preferred treatment for palliation of malignant colonic obstruction (unresectable metastases, unresectable patients): it reduces the rate of stoma, the duration of hospital stay, and morbidity and mortality, and permits rapid initiation of chemotherapy, and then could reduce the medical costs [18, 19].

6.1.2 SEMS Treatment

6.1.2.1 Preparation

General Consideration Before SEMS Insertion

The precise clinical examination should be performed for patient's managements: search for electrolytes imbalances, evaluation of medical comorbidity, investigate the location of obstruction with abdomino-pelvic computed tomography (CT), achieve the locoregional and metastatic staging and identify contraindications (e.g. perforation, small bowel incarceration) to stent insertion. The contraindication for SEMS insertion is intestinal perforation, and additionally peritoneal carcinomatosis and distal margin of tumors close to the anal verge (<5 cm) [18, 19] (Table 6.1). The patients should check-up the pre-anesthesia for medical-surgical consideration in emergency situation like stent insertion complications (perforation, insertion failure). The patients get the intravenous line with fluid therapy and administer with antibiotics for marked dilated colon and complete obstruction. However, antibiotic prophylaxis in obstructed patients undergoing colon stenting is not routine indicated because the risk of post-procedural infections is very low. But, prophylactic antibiotics is used to prevent the incident sepsis or microperforation in case of complete obstruction with marked intestinal dilations because it might be developed during stent insertion procedure [20].

Table 6.1 Contraindications of self-expandable metallic stent (SEMS) insertion

Definite	Clinical signs of peritonitis
	Clinical and radiological signs of perforation or colonic suffering
	Associated small intestine obstruction
Relative	Time required to obtain endoscopic expertise
	Peritoneal carcinomatosis
	Patients undergoing anti-angiogenic therapy or for whom anti-angiogenic treatment is being considered
	Cancer of the lower and middle rectum (less than 3–5 cm from anal verge)

In patients with malignant obstruction, there is little study about bowel preparation before stent placement. However, symptomatic bowel obstruction is a relative contraindication to oral bowel intake of purgatives. Usually patients with complete obstruction have evacuated any fecal material to distal colon from stenosis lesion and bowel purgatives intake is not necessary. An enema is advisable to facilitate the stent placement procedure by cleaning the bowel distal to the stenosis [18].

Prior dilatation and passage through tumor stenosis by large caliber endoscope must be avoided and biopsies for pathologic diagnosis and possible molecular biological analyses (RAS and MSI status) are required for subsequent oncological decisions [19].

For patients with malignant colonic obstruction of proximal colon and potentially curable status, radical resection is recommended as the preferred treatment [18]. However, SEMS insertions have the acceptable clinical and technical success in malignant stenosis located in the proximal colon [21–25]. SEMS insertion is an effective alternative treatment to surgery for palliation of extracolonic malignant obstruction; although technical success and clinical success rates for extracolonic malignancies are slightly inferior to those reported in stenting of primary colonic cancer [26–30].

6.1.2.2 Materials (Instruments) and Techniques

Instruments

The use of a CO_2 inflator is highly suggested during colonic stent insertion: in theory this technique reduces gastrointestinal distension and the risk of perforation and then it induced the patients' tolerance [19]. There were no data about the prevention of risk of complications by inflation with air and CO_2. In the absence of a CO_2 inflator, inflation during progression to the stenosis and during progression to the stenosis and during the implantation of the prosthesis must be as small as possible [19]. A washing pump is useful for facilitating progression to the stenosis [19].

Stent Types

SEMS classified to uncovered or covered according to the presence of meshwork of the stent is bare-wire or covered with polyurethane to prevent tissue ingrowth into the stent. Various types of SEMS are released by many commercial companies (Table 6.2). Most of SEMS are made with wire of Nitinol: a metal alloy of nickel and titanium.

The choice of SEMS is mostly depended on the preference of endoscopists. Covered stent is designed for preventing the tumor ingrowth through the mesh of stent, though it developed the similar number of events between covered and uncovered stents. Surprisingly, it has more frequent event of late migration than uncovered stent. There are no differences of technical success rates, clinical success rates and early complications between covered and uncovered stents. Therefore, most experts recommend that uncovered SEMS is the first choice for the malignant colorectal obstruction in guideline [18, 19]. The appropriate length of SEMS is determined by measured the length of stenosis of obstructive lesion, and then constantly should be at least 3–4 cm longer than the stenosis.

Techniques and Procedure Sequence

SEMS placement is usually performed by using either the through the-scope (TTS) or the over-the-guidewire (OTW) method. Most of all SEMS insertion is done with colonoscope under use of fluoroscopic guidance: TTS method. OTW method is done using fluoroscopic guidance with or without colonoscopic images. The success rates of technical and clinical are comparable between TTS and OTW method [15, 17, 18, 21, 31–34]. Recently most experts recommended that colonic stent placement might be useful under circumstance of combined with endoscope and fluoroscopic guidance (Fig. 6.1).

First step catheterization: The colonoscope was advanced to the obstructive distal site and a guidewire preloaded on the endoscopic retrograde cholangiopancreatography catheter was introduced under endoscopic and fluoroscopic guidance. After passing through the lesion, the

Table 6.2 Variable types of colorectal SEMS (self-expandable metallic stent)

Name	Materials	Types of SEMS	Length (mm)	Diameter (mm)	Company
Niti-s Enteral stent [D-type]	Nitinol	Uncovered	60, 80, 100, 120	18–28	Taewoong Medical
Comvi stent	Nitinol	Covered	60, 80, 100, 120	18–28	Taewoong Medical
Hanarostent	Nitinol	Uncovered	70–170	20, 22, 24	MI Tech
	Nitinol	Covered	60–180	22, 24	
Wallflex Colonic stent	Nitinol	Uncoverd	60, 90, 120	22, 25	Boston Scientific
EGIS Colorectal stent	Nitinol	Uncovered	60, 80, 100, 120	18–30	S&G Biotech
	Nitinol	Covered	60, 80, 100, 120	18–30	
BONASTENT Colorectal	Nitinol	Uncovered	60, 80, 100	22–26	EndoChoice
	Nitinol	Covered	90, 80, 100	22–26	

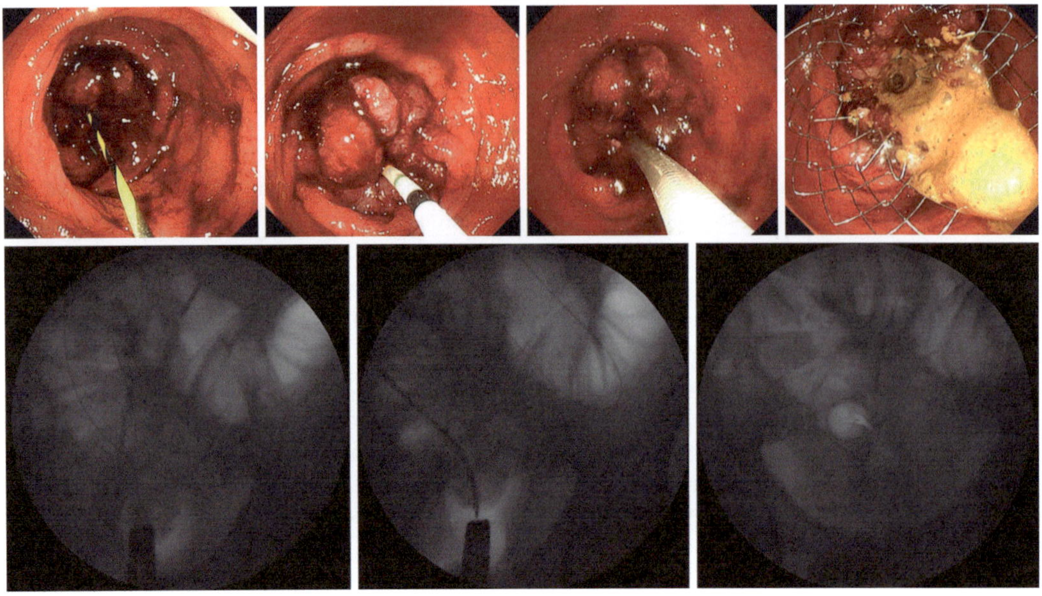

Fig. 6.1 Colonic stent placement is useful under circumstance of combined with endoscope and fluoroscopic guidance in malignant colorectal obstruction

catheter was advanced over the guidewire to the proximal end of the stricture. Second step evaluation of the lesion: The guidewire was removed and a soluble contrast medium was injected to determine the length and morphology of the lesion. Third step insertion of the stent: The catheter was then replaced by the guidewire. SEMS delivery catheter was then advanced through the working channel of the colonoscope over the guidewire until the catheter was positioned across the obstructive site. Final step SEMS deployment: Upon the release of stent delivery catheter, stent deployment began proximally and progressed distally with some static traction forces for preventing proximal migration as monitored by colonoscopy and fluoroscopy. After the deployment of the SEMS, the delivery system and guidewire were removed (Fig. 6.2). The type of inserted SEMS was decided by the endoscopists during the procedure [15].

There are some considerations during catheterization as below. In case of easy positioning of the endoscope in front of the stenosis (left colon, transverse, rectum), the use of flexible catheter with a single or dual channel with long (>450 cm) flexible (or fully flexible) hydrophilic guidewire tip allows the placement of stent TTS under fluoroscopy, combining safety and efficiency [19]. In difficult catheterization, the stenosis is lateralized, or angular, or the position of the endoscope is unstable (recto-sigmoid colon, sigmoid colon, splenic and hepatic flexures), the stenosis is right or the stenosis is tortuous. These situations require the help of a pre-curved adjustable catheter, or a rotary sphincterotome, and the use of "J" guide wire technique, or a thinner guide wire (0.018 or 0.025 in.) [19]. The materials and techniques used in this situation are the same as those used for endoscopic retrograde cholangio-pancreatography (ERCP). The use of biliopancreatic catheterization materials and long non-traumatic hydrophilic guides is advocated [19].

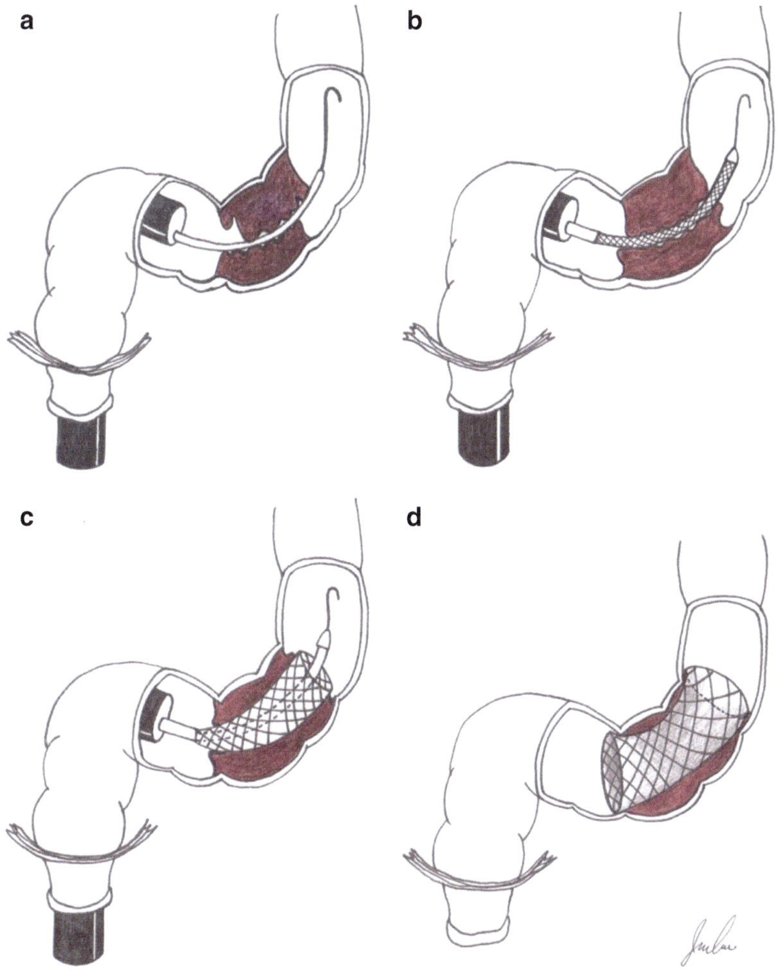

Fig. 6.2 The Schematic sequence of SEMS placement. (**a**) The colonoscope was advanced to the obstructive distal site and a guidewire preloaded on the endoscopic retrograde cholangiopancreatography catheter was introduced under endoscopic and fluoroscopic guidance. After passing through the lesion, the catheter was advanced over the guidewire to the proximal end of the stricture. (**b**) The guidewire was removed and a soluble contrast medium was injected to determine the length and morphology of the lesion. The catheter was then replaced by the guidewire. (**c**) SEMS delivery catheter was then advanced through the working channel of the colonoscope over the guidewire until the catheter was positioned across the obstructive site. (**d**) Upon the release of stent delivery catheter, stent deployment began proximally and progressed distally with some static traction forces for preventing proximal migration as monitored by colonoscopy and fluoroscopy. After the deployment of the SEMS, the delivery system and guidewire were removed

6.1.3 Clinical Consideration After SEMS Insertion

6.1.3.1 Complication

Early complications evaluated between 2 and 7 days after SEMS insertion. The serious complications of SEMS insertion are very good with an immediate mortality rate of below 1% in most published studies (average 0.6%) [16–19, 35–49]. SEMS insertion caused early complications such as perforation (0–12.8%), migration (0–13%), and less frequently bleeding (0–3.7%) [18, 19]. Last two complications are managed by conservative cares with colonoscopy. However, perforation usually need to emergent surgical treatment and is the most common cause of early mortality. Perforation is also bad prognosis factors of oncologic outcomes.

Late complication might be related to the results at 30 or 7 days [15, 39, 50]. The 30 days mortality rate was 9% with half of the deaths related to poor prognosis of cancer [19]. The late complications occurred 16–31% of patients [15, 22]. The rate of late perforations ranged from 1 to 7% [19]. The risk factors of late perforation are associated with the type of stent use, the presence of peritoneal carcinomatosis, and chemotherapy including anti-angiogenic therapy [15, 18, 19, 22, 51]. The suspected mechanism may be that inhibition of vascular endothelial growth factor (VEGF) results in tissue hypoxia, which leads to tissue necrosis and perforation at the tumor site [15]. Therefore, we should be considered the increased risk of perforation for patients administered with chemotherapy after SEMS insertion. However, patients who have undergone stenting for palliation could be safely treated with chemotherapy without anti-angiogenic agents (bevacizumav, aflibercept and regorafenib) If a patient is considered for chemotherapeutic treatment with anti-angiogenic agents, it is not recommended to use palliative SEMS insertion in high risk of patients with perforation [18]. Baron et al. proposed that stent-related perforation may result from different causes: (a) guidewire or catheter malpositioning; (b) dilation of stricture before or after stent placement; (c) stent-induced perforation (tumor and non-tumor local perforation); and (d) proximal colonic distension because of inadequate colonic decompression or excessive air insufflation [18, 52]. The rate of late migration ranged from 1.0 to 12.5% and this risk is closely related with the types of stent: covered stent occupied the most proportion of late event and also small diameter SEMS (<24 mm) [15, 18, 53, 54]. Some studies reported that chemotherapy might be associated with late migration of SEMS by the mechanism of tumor shrinkage [18, 31, 50]. Stent re-obstruction occurred due to tumor in/overgrowth and also during the long-term follow up period. The use of uncovered SEMS is risk factor for tumor ingrowth [44]. Suh et al. presented that less than 70% stent expansion within first 48 h is predictive marker for estimating the occurrence of re-obstruction [55]. Both migration and re-obstruction can be managed with colonoscopic methods. Stent replacement and stent reopening by a stent-in-stent have been reported as first choice in the majority of studies, with satisfactory outcomes (clinical success rates 75–86%) [15, 18, 22, 56].

After SEMS insertion, we should evaluate the immediate and late complications like as careful and precise interview of abdomen symptoms and physical examination of peritonitis, abdomen supine and erection or simple abdomen for kidney ureter and bladder (KUB). Also, the serial assessment for regression of obstructive symptoms and signs should be performed within 48 h after SEMS insertion. The symptoms and signs of obstruction are improved after SEMS insertion and then oral intake slowly try with sips of water. There are no other symptoms and signs after water intakes, sequential diet try to start with soft diet like low residual diet. If fecal material is hard consistency in patients with distal obstruction, stool softener should be prescribed for preventing stool impaction.

Several studies reported that the median patency duration of palliative SEMS was 106 days (range 68–288 days) [14–16, 18, 57]. Although consensus follow up schedule for SEMS is not existed, it might be performed concordance with regular surveillance for colorectal cancer. However, if the patients with SEMS have symptoms and signs of obstruction, we should be investigated the complications.

Some studies present that synchronous colorectal tumors occur in 3–4% of patients with colorectal cancer [58–60]. Preoperative CT colonography and colonoscopy through the stent appear feasible and safe in malignant colorectal obstruction and there are no data discourage their use in some studies [61–64].

There are many studies about the clinical efficacy of SEMS insertion for patients with malignant colorectal obstruction. SEMS placement gains the better short-term outcomes to decompress obstructive symptoms compared with emergent surgery. SEMS insertion additionally can avoid the emergent surgery with stoma creation which has the high morbidity and mortality.

6.2 Ballooning for Benign Colorectal Strictures

6.2.1 Introduction

The various causes of colonic strictures includes inflammatory bowel disease (Crohn's and ulcerative colitis), anastomotic leakages, ischemia, malignancy, radiation injury, nonsteroidal anti-inflammatory drugs (NSAIDs), and as a consequence of diverticulitis [65]. The etiology-specific prevalence of colonic strictures is not known for all of these conditions but is as high as 13.5% in Crohn's disease [65]. Colorectal strictures induced by non-malignant conditions were managed with various treatment modalities, especially balloon dilatation. Ballooning reduces the symptoms and signs of benign strictures like constipation, abdominal pain and vomiting and also prevents the secondary perforation induced strictures. Balloon dilatation is the simple and easily used modality and relatively safe and effective.

6.2.2 Indications

6.2.2.1 Anastomotic Strictures

Colonic anastomosis strictures develops up to 22% of patients following colon resection and anastomosis [66]. The reasons of strictures are inappropriate anastomosis, anastomotic leakages, ischemia, pre- or post-radiation treatment, infectious diseases and anastomotic dehiscence. Strictures dilation could be managed using balloon dilators with or without electrical devices. Pucciarelli et al. presented that factors associated with a successful outcomes to dilation were high level anastomosis (>8 cm from anal verge), no radiation treatment, minimal or no dehiscence, no neoplastic recurrence, simple stricture shapes, and short stenosis (<1 cm) and combination of radiotherapy, local neoplastic recurrence, and large dehiscence was related with failure of a single dilation of nearly 100% [67]. If anastomotic stricture is membranous types, it is very good response to ballooning. However, transmural or concentric strictures are less responsive to endoscopic balloon treatment.

6.2.2.2 Inflammatory Bowel Diseases

Intestinal strictures more frequently occurred in Crohn's disease (CD) than ulcerative colitis and it developed at every site like colon, small intestine and duodenum. Strictures of CD are the critical important complications which make patients admit the hospital and induced subocclusive symptoms to patients. In formers times, strictures induced CD were managed by operation. However, recently, endoscopic balloon dilatation was performed with considering the recurrence of CD and morbidity of operation. Systematic review presented that endoscopic dilatation initially achieved technical success in 86% of stricture cases and long term clinical efficacy is up to 58% of the patients [68]. Efficacies of endoscopic ballooning for strictures of CD reported were mostly favorable; however, long term clinical outcomes were variable: the recurrence ranged from 13 to 100% and then we should be undergone repeated endoscopic ballooning [69–72]. Feres et al. represented that 42% of CD with recurrent stricture are finally taken the operation after ballooning [73]. After balloon dilatation, continuous treatment for CD should be continued for preventing recurrence. The risk factor of stricture recurrence is associated with long segment of stricture; a stricture length (≤4 cm) was associated with a surgery free outcome [68].

6.2.3 Preparation and Contraindication

Before endoscopic ballooning dilatation abdomen pelvic CT should be taken for precise evaluation of the site, length, and morphology of strictures. The contraindication is active inflammation like abscess of CD, long length segment of stricture and fistula of CD due to complication of perforation and re-operation needed. In rectum, endoscopic ultrasound and MRI also helpful evaluation methods but it is not inevitable. Bowel preparation is done depends on the severity of stricture; if there is no symptoms of complete obstruction, routine bowel preparation should be taken and patients with partial or complete obstruction take the enema. Also, sedation was administered as necessary depending on patient tolerance. The diameter of balloon was first chosen the larger size than the diameter of stricture and then changed more big size balloon than first size. There are no definite final size of balloon diameter, duration time of balloon inflation, and the number of repeated balloon inflation. It depends on the severity of stricture. Most of all TTS balloons were used for dilatation with or without under the fluoroscopic guidance. Dilation was performed with balloons ranging in diameter from 18 to 25 mm [68].

6.2.4 Insertion Technique

Distal site of the stricture is identified with standard colonoscope. And then a guidewire preloaded on the catheter was introduced to pass through the stricture lesion and the catheter was advanced over the guidewire to the proximal end of the stricture. The guidewire was removed and a soluble contrast medium was injected to determine the length and morphology of the lesion. The catheter was then replaced by the guidewire. Balloon catheter was then advanced through the working channel of the endoscope over the guidewire until the balloon catheter passed 2–3 cm beyond the proximal stricture site. The balloon was filled with distilled water or water soluble contrast dye to maintain the outer diameter at optimal size and was kept in the same position for a period of 5 min using the standard inflation pressure suggested by manufacturer; this step was repeated again with different balloon catheter depends on the stricture status after balloon dilation until endoscope passed through the stricture.

6.2.5 Results After Ballooning Procedure

The complications also occurred like perforation, bleeding, abdomen pain and infection after ballooning. Gustavsson et al. reported the complications of ballooning that perforation is 1.4%, massive bleeding is 1%, and pain and infection is 1.5% [74]. Therefore, after ballooning, we should evaluate the patient with abdomen supine and erection or chest X-ray and close physical examination when patients complain abdominal pain.

The favorable clinical factors are initial technical success, short segment of stricture, smoking and absence of ulcer in stricture [75]. Thienpont et al., however, suggested that disease activity, CRP and endoscopic severity did not affect the clinical outcomes [76].

Endoscopic ballooning is a relatively feasible and effective treatment modality in anastomotic strictures and strictures of inflammatory bowel disease (esp. Crohn's disease).

References

1. Deans GT, Krukowski ZH, Irwin ST. Malignant obstruction of the left colon. Br J Surg. 1994;81:1270–6.
2. Iversen LH, Bulow S, Christensen IJ, et al. Postoperative medical complications are the main cause of early death after emergency surgery for colonic cancer. Br J Surg. 2008;95:1012–9.
3. Law WL, Choi HK, Chu KW. Comparison of stenting with emergency surgery as palliative treatment for obstructing primary left-sided colorectal cancer. Br J Surg. 2003;90:1429–33.
4. Martinez-Santos C, Lobato RF, Fradejas JM, et al. Self-expandable stent before elective surgery vs. emergency surgery for the treatment of malignant colorectal obstructions: comparison of primary anastomosis and morbidity rates. Dis Colon Rectum. 2002;45:401–6.
5. Saida Y, Sumiyama Y, Nagao J, et al. Long-term prognosis of preoperative "bridge to surgery" expandable metallic stent insertion for obstructive colorectal cancer: comparison with emergency operation. Dis Colon Rectum. 2003;46:S44–9.
6. Smothers L, Hynan L, Fleming J, et al. Emergency surgery for colon carcinoma. Dis Colon Rectum. 2003;46:24–30.
7. Nagula S, Ishill N, Nash C, et al. Quality of life and symptom control after stent placement or surgical palliation of malignant colorectal obstruction. J Am Coll Surg. 2010;210:45–53.
8. Dohmoto M. New method-endoscopic implantation of rectal stent in palliative treatment of malignant stenosis. Endosc Dig. 1991;3:1507–12.
9. Spinelli P, Dal Fante M, Mancini A. Self-expanding mesh stent for endoscopic palliation of rectal obstructing tumors: a preliminary report. Surg Endosc. 1992;6:72–4.
10. Camunez F, Echenagusia A, Simo G, et al. Malignant colorectal obstruction treated by means of self-expanding metallic stents: effectiveness before surgery and in palliation. Radiology. 2000;216:492–7.

11. Cole SJ, Boorman P, Osman HS, et al. Endoluminal stenting for relief of colonic obstruction is safe and effective. Color Dis. 2000;2:282–7.
12. de Gregorio MA, Mainar A, Tejero E, et al. Acute colorectal obstruction: stent placement for palliative treatment–results of a multicenter study. Radiology. 1998;209:117–20.
13. Lee HJ, Hong SP, Cheon JH, et al. Long-term outcome of palliative therapy for malignant colorectal obstruction in patients with unresectable metastatic colorectal cancers: endoscopic stenting versus surgery. Gastrointest Endosc. 2011;73:535–42.
14. Park JK, Lee MS, Ko BM, et al. Outcome of palliative self-expanding metal stent placement in malignant colorectal obstruction according to stent type and manufacturer. Surg Endosc. 2011;25:1293–9.
15. Kim BC, Han KS, Hong CW, et al. Clinical outcomes of palliative self-expanding metallic stents in patients with malignant colorectal obstruction. J Dig Dis. 2012;13:258–66.
16. Watt AM, Faragher IG, Griffin TT, et al. Self-expanding metallic stents for relieving malignant colorectal obstruction: a systematic review. Ann Surg. 2007;246:24–30.
17. Sebastian S, Johnston S, Geoghegan T, et al. Pooled analysis of the efficacy and safety of self-expanding metal stenting in malignant colorectal obstruction. Am J Gastroenterol. 2004;99:2051–7.
18. van Hooft JE, van Halsema EE, Vanbiervliet G, et al. Self-expandable metal stents for obstructing colonic and extracolonic cancer: European Society of Gastrointestinal Endoscopy (ESGE) Clinical Guideline. Endoscopy. 2014;46:990–1053.
19. Endoscopy and Cancer Committee of the French Society of Digestive Endoscopy, the French Federation of Digestive Oncology. Place of colorectal stents in therapeutic management of malignant large bowel obstructions. Endoscopy. 2014;46:546–52.
20. Keymling M. Colorectal stenting. Endoscopy. 2003;35:234–8.
21. Geraghty J, Sarkar S, Cox T, et al. Management of large bowel obstruction with self-expanding metal stents. A multicentre retrospective study of factors determining outcome. Color Dis. 2014;16:476–83.
22. Yoon JY, Jung YS, Hong SP, et al. Clinical outcomes and risk factors for technical and clinical failures of self-expandable metal stent insertion for malignant colorectal obstruction. Gastrointest Endosc. 2011;74:858–68.
23. Yao LQ, Zhong YS, Xu MD, et al. Self-expanding metallic stents drainage for acute proximal colon obstruction. World J Gastroenterol. 2011;17:3342–6.
24. Cho YK, Kim SW, Lee BI, et al. Clinical outcome of self-expandable metal stent placement in the management of malignant proximal colon obstruction. Gut Liver. 2011;5:165–70.
25. Repici A, Adler DG, Gibbs CM, et al. Stenting of the proximal colon in patients with malignant large bowel obstruction: techniques and outcomes. Gastrointest Endosc. 2007;66:940–4.
26. Moon SJ, Kim SW, Lee BI, et al. Palliative stent for malignant colonic obstruction by extracolonic malignancy: a comparison with colorectal cancer. Dig Dis Sci. 2014;59:1891–7.
27. Kim JY, Kim SG, Im JP, et al. Comparison of treatment outcomes of endoscopic stenting for colonic and extracolonic malignant obstruction. Surg Endosc. 2013;27:272–7.
28. Kim BK, Hong SP, Heo HM, et al. Endoscopic stenting is not as effective for palliation of colorectal obstruction in patients with advanced gastric cancer as emergency surgery. Gastrointest Endosc. 2012;75:294–301.
29. Keswani RN, Azar RR, Edmundowicz SA, et al. Stenting for malignant colonic obstruction: a comparison of efficacy and complications in colonic versus extracolonic malignancy. Gastrointest Endosc. 2009;69:675–80.
30. Shin SJ, Kim TI, Kim BC, et al. Clinical application of self-expandable metallic stent for treatment of colorectal obstruction caused by extrinsic invasive tumors. Dis Colon Rectum. 2008;51:578–83.
31. Kim JH, Song HY, Li YD, et al. Dual-design expandable colorectal stent for malignant colorectal obstruction: comparison of flared ends and bent ends. AJR Am J Roentgenol. 2009;193:248–54.
32. Kim SY, Kwon SH, Oh JH. Radiologic placement of uncovered stents for the treatment of malignant colorectal obstruction. J Vasc Interv Radiol. 2010;21:1244–9.
33. Selinger CP, Ramesh J, Martin DF. Long-term success of colonic stent insertion is influenced by indication but not by length of stent or site of obstruction. Int J Color Dis. 2011;26:215–8.
34. Kim JW, Jeong JB, Lee KL, et al. Comparison of clinical outcomes between endoscopic and radiologic placement of self-expandable metal stent in patients with malignant colorectal obstruction. Korean J Gastroenterol. 2013;61:22–9.
35. Khot UP, Lang AW, Murali K, et al. Systematic review of the efficacy and safety of colorectal stents. Br J Surg. 2002;89:1096–102.
36. Tilney HS, Lovegrove RE, Purkayastha S, et al. Comparison of colonic stenting and open surgery for malignant large bowel obstruction. Surg Endosc. 2007;21:225–33.
37. Cheung HY, Chung CC, Tsang WW, et al. Endolaparoscopic approach vs conventional open surgery in the treatment of obstructing left-sided colon cancer: a randomized controlled trial. Arch Surg. 2009;144:1127–32.
38. Alcantara M, Serra-Aracil X, Falco J, et al. Prospective, controlled, randomized study of intraoperative colonic lavage versus stent placement in obstructive left-sided colonic cancer. World J Surg. 2011;35:1904–10.
39. Meisner S, Gonzalez-Huix F, Vandervoort JG, et al. Self-expandable metal stents for relieving malignant colorectal obstruction: short-term safety and efficacy within 30 days of stent procedure in 447 patients. Gastrointest Endosc. 2011;74:876–84.

40. Pirlet IA, Slim K, Kwiatkowski F, et al. Emergency preoperative stenting versus surgery for acute left-sided malignant colonic obstruction: a multicenter randomized controlled trial. Surg Endosc. 2011;25:1814–21.
41. van Hooft JE, Bemelman WA, Oldenburg B, et al. Colonic stenting versus emergency surgery for acute left-sided malignant colonic obstruction: a multicentre randomised trial. Lancet Oncol. 2011;12:344–52.
42. Ho KS, Quah HM, Lim JF, et al. Endoscopic stenting and elective surgery versus emergency surgery for left-sided malignant colonic obstruction: a prospective randomized trial. Int J Color Dis. 2012;27:355–62.
43. Tan CJ, Dasari BV, Gardiner K. Systematic review and meta-analysis of randomized clinical trials of self-expanding metallic stents as a bridge to surgery versus emergency surgery for malignant left-sided large bowel obstruction. Br J Surg. 2012;99:469–76.
44. Zhang Y, Shi J, Shi B, et al. Self-expanding metallic stent as a bridge to surgery versus emergency surgery for obstructive colorectal cancer: a meta-analysis. Surg Endosc. 2012;26:110–9.
45. Cennamo V, Luigiano C, Coccolini F, et al. Meta-analysis of randomized trials comparing endoscopic stenting and surgical decompression for colorectal cancer obstruction. Int J Color Dis. 2013;28:855–63.
46. Cirocchi R, Farinella E, Trastulli S, et al. Safety and efficacy of endoscopic colonic stenting as a bridge to surgery in the management of intestinal obstruction due to left colon and rectal cancer: a systematic review and meta-analysis. Surg Oncol. 2013;22:14–21.
47. De Ceglie A, Filiberti R, Baron TH, et al. A meta-analysis of endoscopic stenting as bridge to surgery versus emergency surgery for left-sided colorectal cancer obstruction. Crit Rev Oncol Hematol. 2013;88:387–403.
48. Ghazal AH, El-Shazly WG, Bessa SS, et al. Colonic endolumenal stenting devices and elective surgery versus emergency subtotal/total colectomy in the management of malignant obstructed left colon carcinoma. J Gastrointest Surg. 2013;17:1123–9.
49. Huang X, Lv B, Zhang S, et al. Preoperative colonic stents versus emergency surgery for acute left-sided malignant colonic obstruction: a meta-analysis. J Gastrointest Surg. 2014;18:584–91.
50. Fernandez-Esparrach G, Bordas JM, Giraldez MD, et al. Severe complications limit long-term clinical success of self-expanding metal stents in patients with obstructive colorectal cancer. Am J Gastroenterol. 2010;105:1087–93.
51. van Hooft JE, Fockens P, Marinelli AW, et al. Early closure of a multicenter randomized clinical trial of endoscopic stenting versus surgery for stage IV left-sided colorectal cancer. Endoscopy. 2008;40:184–91.
52. Baron TH, Wong Kee Song LM, Repici A. Role of self-expandable stents for patients with colon cancer (with videos). Gastrointest Endosc. 2012;75:653–62.
53. Small AJ, Coelho-Prabhu N, Baron TH. Endoscopic placement of self-expandable metal stents for malignant colonic obstruction: long-term outcomes and complication factors. Gastrointest Endosc. 2010;71:560–72.
54. Manes G, de Bellis M, Fuccio L, et al. Endoscopic palliation in patients with incurable malignant colorectal obstruction by means of self-expanding metal stent: analysis of results and predictors of outcomes in a large multicenter series. Arch Surg. 2011;146:1157–62.
55. Suh JP, Kim SW, Cho YK, et al. Effectiveness of stent placement for palliative treatment in malignant colorectal obstruction and predictive factors for stent occlusion. Surg Endosc. 2010;24:400–6.
56. Yoon JY, Jung YS, Hong SP, et al. Outcomes of secondary stent-in-stent self-expandable metal stent insertion for malignant colorectal obstruction. Gastrointest Endosc. 2011;74:625–33.
57. Cheung DY, Kim JY, Hong SP, et al. Outcome and safety of self-expandable metallic stents for malignant colon obstruction: a Korean multicenter randomized prospective study. Surg Endosc. 2012;26:3106–13.
58. Kodeda K, Nathanaelsson L, Jung B, et al. Population-based data from the Swedish Colon Cancer Registry. Br J Surg. 2013;100:1100–7.
59. Mulder SA, Kranse R, Damhuis RA, et al. Prevalence and prognosis of synchronous colorectal cancer: a Dutch population-based study. Cancer Epidemiol. 2011;35:442–7.
60. Latournerie M, Jooste V, Cottet V, et al. Epidemiology and prognosis of synchronous colorectal cancers. Br J Surg. 2008;95:1528–33.
61. Lim SG, Lee KJ, Suh KW, et al. Preoperative colonoscopy for detection of synchronous neoplasms after insertion of self-expandable metal stents in occlusive colorectal cancer: comparison of covered and uncovered stents. Gut Liver. 2013;7:311–6.
62. Park SH, Lee JH, Lee SS, et al. CT colonography for detection and characterisation of synchronous proximal colonic lesions in patients with stenosing colorectal cancer. Gut. 2012;61:1716–22.
63. Cha EY, Park SH, Lee SS, et al. CT colonography after metallic stent placement for acute malignant colonic obstruction. Radiology. 2010;254:774–82.
64. Vitale MA, Villotti G, d'Alba L, et al. Preoperative colonoscopy after self-expandable metallic stent placement in patients with acute neoplastic colon obstruction. Gastrointest Endosc. 2006;63:814–9.
65. Lemberg B, Vargo JJ. Balloon dilation of colonic strictures. Am J Gastroenterol. 2007;102:2123–5.
66. Geller A, Gal E. Dilation of benign strictures following low anterior resection using Savary-Gilliard bougies. Endoscopic treatment of benign anastomotic colorectal stenosis with electrocautery. Gastrointest Endosc. 2001;54:277–9.
67. Pucciarelli S, Toppan P, Pilati PL, et al. Efficacy of dilatations for anastomotic colorectal stenoses: prognostic factors. Int J Color Dis. 1994;9:149–52.
68. Hassan C, Zullo A, De Francesco V, et al. Systematic review: endoscopic dilatation in Crohn's disease. Aliment Pharmacol Ther. 2007;26:1457–64.

69. Blomberg B, Rolny P, Jarnerot G. Endoscopic treatment of anastomotic strictures in Crohn's disease. Endoscopy. 1991;23:195–8.
70. Couckuyt H, Gevers AM, Coremans G, et al. Efficacy and safety of hydrostatic balloon dilatation of ileocolonic Crohn's strictures: a prospective longterm analysis. Gut. 1995;36:577–80.
71. Thomas-Gibson S, Brooker JC, Hayward CM, et al. Colonoscopic balloon dilation of Crohn's strictures: a review of long-term outcomes. Eur J Gastroenterol Hepatol. 2003;15:485–8.
72. Singh VV, Draganov P, Valentine J. Efficacy and safety of endoscopic balloon dilation of symptomatic upper and lower gastrointestinal Crohn's disease strictures. J Clin Gastroenterol. 2005;39:284–90.
73. Feres M, Gursky LC, Faveri M, et al. Clinical and microbiological benefits of strict supragingival plaque control as part of the active phase of periodontal therapy. J Clin Periodontol. 2009;36:857–67.
74. Gustavsson A, Magnuson A, Blomberg B, et al. Endoscopic dilation is an efficacious and safe treatment of intestinal strictures in Crohn's disease. Aliment Pharmacol Ther. 2012;36:151–8.
75. Hoffmann JC, Heller F, Faiss S, et al. Through the endoscope balloon dilation of ileocolonic strictures: prognostic factors, complications, and effectiveness. Int J Color Dis. 2008;23:689–96.
76. Thienpont C, D'Hoore A, Vermeire S, et al. Long-term outcome of endoscopic dilatation in patients with Crohn's disease is not affected by disease activity or medical therapy. Gut. 2010;59:320–4.

Index

D.K. Sohn (ed.), *Practice and Principles in Therapeutic Colonoscopy*,
https://doi.org/10.1007/978-3-662-46552-3

MIX
Papier aus verantwortungsvollen Quellen
Paper from responsible sources
FSC® C105338

If you have any concerns about our products,
you can contact us on
ProductSafety@springernature.com

In case Publisher is established outside the EU,
the EU authorized representative is:
Springer Nature Customer Service Center GmbH
Europaplatz 3, 69115 Heidelberg, Germany

Printed by Libri Plureos GmbH
in Hamburg, Germany